RESOLVING SEXUAL ISSUES

with Creative Mindpower Techniques

RESOLVING SEXUAL ISSUES
with Creative Mindpower Techniques

THE DIFINITIVE SELF-HELP SELF-HYPNOSIS GUIDE

Dr. Frank W. Lea, DD,
Dip.NLP(Master Practitioner),
RPHH, APHP

Order this book online at www.trafford.com
or email orders@trafford.com

Most Trafford titles are also available at major online book retailers.

Printed in the United States of America.

ISBN: 978-1-4269-5121-3 (sc)
ISBN: 978-1-4269-5120-6 (e)

Trafford rev. 01/27/2014

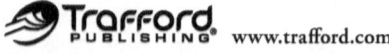 www.trafford.com

North America & International
toll-free: 1 888 232 4444 (USA & Canada)
fax: 812 355 4082

A very well written and insightful book.

Frank manages to capture and make clear how our minds can work with or against us in cases of illness and recovery, this is definitely something every serious therapist should have on their bookshelf!

Nick Davies (Owner and Director)
Warwickshire School of Hypnotherapy
www.WSOH.co.uk

Frank, I am truly thankful for your treatment, I have a new and resounding commitment to the current projects in my life. Thank you
Paul J. Soden, www.qlifetraining.com

What an amazing therapist. Frank helped me eliminate trauma I had carried for two years, I can't say enough wonderful things about him.

Jane F. – USA

Frank Lea showed us his Creative Mind Therapy for both myself in 2004 and my daughter this year, 2005, the evening before we took our Driving Test. Both of us are born worriers and think negative thoughts especially when the word 'TEST' is involved and could only think on the lines of "I am not going to pass". The Therapy solved all that negativity and was worth every penny, for only one 1 hour session, going home we both felt this isn't going to work, on getting up the next day, the actual fear had left and we both felt determined to pass, guess what, we did. I could not recommend this therapy more highly and would not hesitate to use it again if the need arose.

A very grateful client.

Dear Frank,

Just a few words to let you know how I have been getting on after my session with you back in April when you helped me with my fear of heights and skiing. I have just got back from holiday in Chamonix in the French Alps. I went up several mountains in cable cars and also used the chair lift. I was comfortable and certainly not panicking. I felt for the first time that I was in control and could handle it. I was able to put my fear of heights in place and not let it stop me doing what I wanted to do. The results so far are amazing and I would like to thank you. My husband is extremely pleased and happy for me and we are looking forward to getting on the slopes with our sons. I have been in touch with the Phobics Society to let them know of my wonderful experience.

Many, many thanks. Margaret.

Sufferered from OCD 5 yrs. Doctors and psychiatrists and drugs no help: Date: Tue,

27 Nov 2007 10:51:27

From: Mick

To: actpublications@yahoo.co.uk Hello Frank. Just to let you know that I have seen a dramatic Just to let you know that I have seen a dramatic improvement in my conditions since my session, I no longer feel the need further treatment. Thanks for your help. Regards, Mick Henderson

FOREWORD
BY Dr. JONATHAN ROYLE

Dear Reader,

I am excited to have been asked to write the foreword for this truly life-changing book, as you will see on my website <u>www.magicguru.com</u> I have been involved in the Personal Development, Self-Help and Psychological Healing arenas for over 21+ years to date and indeed these days I act as an advisor and consultant for some of the biggest names in the field.

I have known Dr. Frank W. Lea, DD, Dip.NLP(Master Practitioner), RPHH, APHP for many years now and I have absolutely no doubts about his knowledge and skills in matters of the mind and healing and his genuine desire to help people to change and improve their lives and be free of any negative influence that may be holding them back from achieving their true potential.

There are many self-healing books around but I believe this one to be unique in that it contains simple yet powerful techniques for addressing sexual issues, sexuality and sexual problems, particularly with reference to victims of rape and sexual abuse.

Reading this book will give you amazing insight into the workings of the mind and how to use that knowledge to easily and safely understand and overcome your own issues and to help others who have similar issues.

Uniquely for this kind of publication you will find the author, Dr. Frank W. Lea, DD, Dip.NLP(Master Practitioner), RPHH, APHP, easily accessible should you need help or explanation on any aspect of these writings.

So, dear reader, pick up this book and take your first step to achieving the freedom and relief you deserve.

My very best wishes to you
Dr. Jonathan Royle
www.magicguru.com

ACKNOWLEDGEMENTS

I wish to thank Yvonne Oswald, author of *Every Word Has Power* for encouraging me to write this book and its sister book, *Creative Mindpower Techniques to Heal Yourself and Others,* which deals with resolving a huge range of emotional and psychological issues and problems including many bodily conditions. Her support and advice during my work has been invaluable.

Also I wish to thank Dr. Jonathan Royle for his teachings in stage hypnosis which greatly improved my expertise and success as a hypnotherapist.

My first tutor John Howard and later tutors Paul McKenna and Richard Bandler for their invaluable training in hypnosis and neuro linguistic programming, all of which contributed to the development of my own Creative Mindpower Techniques.

Not forgetting all my many hundreds of clients from whom I learnt so much and gained such huge satisfaction from successfully helping them resolve their issues.

HOW IT ALL STARTED

Many years ago a member of my family was diagnosed with a very rare, painful and debilitating complaint which only a few medical professionals knew much about, and no cure was known nor has since been discovered. In addition to this she also suffered from Irritable Bowel Syndrome and Wheat Intolerance. She coped with this stoically for many years.

One fortunate day I spotted a small advertisement offering training in hypnotherapy with a promise that a lucrative and satisfying career was a distinct possibility.

As I had spent many years studying and practicing martial arts I already knew that a great deal of the power of martial arts came from the mind rather than just physical strength and ability. Because of this the idea of hypnosis struck me as possibly providing the means to help my family member through utilising the power of her mind, particularly because the slightest stress always aggravated her condition, so it was obvious to me that because stress was definitely a state of mind and also contributed to the Irritable Bowel Syndrome hypnosis could be a way to ease the stress and alleviate the condition. With this motivation I applied for the course.

This particular course was expected to take up to two years to complete (unlike today where trainers think two or three days` training is sufficient). Amazingly to me, I discovered I had a natural tendency towards hypnotherapy and easily assimilated the knowledge and skills involved. As a result I completed the course in six months and passed the exam with a 94% marking.

Using my new found skills I`m happy to say that I successfully relieved the lady mentioned of her Irritable Bowel Syndrome which led to a reduction in the problem with wheat intolerance. However, I have to admit I have not been wholly successful with the rare condition but have helped reduce its impact far more than the medical people had been able to do to the extent that they asked how this was done because they noticed the change in her condition, since then they utilise the method I showed them to help their other patients.

At a later time I also used my knowledge and skills to help the same lady when she was diagnose with breast cancer – no, I was not able to cure the cancer, at that time I didn`t know how to approach such a task, though I do now. I was, however, able to help her cope with the tremendous emotional and mental trauma (which we know everyone diagnosed with cancer suffers) and was able to help her approach the surgery she needed in a calm and positive manner. Pleasingly the surgeon commented on her state of mind and positive reaction to the surgery, acknowledging that the success of the operation and subsequent speedy recovery was definitely enhanced by it. Happily I have since been able to help many people prior to operations in this way.

Though originally my intention to learn hypnotherapy was purely to help the lady mentioned and not as a career in its own right I derived so much satisfaction from helping people and witnessing the amazing results of hypnotherapy that it did become my main career. Now that I am getting on in years this book is my endeavour to pass on my skills and knowledge so that others can enjoy the satisfaction of healing themselves and other people and, if you like, carrying on the good work, or passing on the good news.

INTRODUCTION

Please note that while this book deals with sexuality and sexual problems it is not written for fun or any kind of sexual enjoyment. It is information vital to those who suffer from sexual problems, are confused about their sexuality or are the victims of sexual abuse. It is aimed at giving insight into how sexualities and sexual inclinations are formed and offers safe and effective ways of dealing with them and includes self-help and understanding for victims of rape and sexual abuse.

Every journey begins with one step and you have taken the first step on an amazing journey to become your own therapist and become free of anything that is less than satisfying in your life and once you have mastered these simple yet powerful techniques you will be able to apply them to help others, in fact you may even decide to take things further and become a professional therapist. Nothing can be more satisfying than knowing you have helped someone change their life for the better and consequently the lives of those around them, for instance, a recent client who, as a result of being abused as a child was unable to have a normal relationship. It is so good to receive a letter to say she is now about to be married – her life and the lives of her husband to be, family and friends is so full of happiness now, and to know that I have played a part in bringing about so much joy is a feeling that very few other careers can achieve.

Dr. Frank W. Lea, DD,
Dip.NLP(Master Practitioner), RPHH, APHP

WHAT HYPNOSIS IS AND WHAT IT CAN ACHIEVE

The terms hypnosis and hypnotherapist are familiar to most people but new to others so the question is often asked "what is hypnosis?" To answer this it helps to describe the work of the hypnotherapist. Originally hypnotherapy was, and often still is, a suggestion based therapy where some concept, idea or suggestion is put forward to the client. This form of therapy is particularly useful to help a person stop smoking for instance.

What *is* hypnotherapy? As with other therapies, hypnotherapy is used to heal, the one unique and vital factor of difference is that hypnotherapy is directed at healing through the power of the subconscious mind, the supreme human bodily programme. In this way it becomes possible to not only treat the mind itself but the entire bodily system in a natural and safe way. This is possible because no part of the body can function without the mind and no part can perform efficiently and properly if the mind fails to completely fulfil its functions relative to that part.

Hypnotherapy is conducted with the subject in the natural state of hypnosis which gives the therapist direct access to the subconscious mind. It is the subconscious mind that governs us and makes us the personality we are and causes us to react in the way that we do, therefore if we are reacting or behaving in a way that is detrimental to us we can change that just like deleting some unwanted programme from a computer and installing a new and better one. Hypnotherapy is not concerned with disease and general illness though it can assist conventional medicine by stimulating the subject's immune system.

Hypnosis should not be used to replace conventional medicine, rather it should go hand in hand with it for the simple reason that should the subject's condition be a symptom of the mind state and the therapist brings about the relief of that state the condition will be resolved in any case.

Regarding the status of hypnotherapy, whether it is an alternative or complimentary therapy I suggest the answer is neither. The hypnotherapist is the only practitioner specialising through hypnosis, therefore it can be considered a separate branch of medicine. Because of the uniqueness of hypnotherapeutic approach and the fact that it is directed at treating the most significant organ of the human body, hypnotherapy must ultimately become recognised as of equal if not more importance than other medical approaches.

Hypnosis can be used to treat a very wide range of conditions, commonly neurotic ones, but also those that appear to be non-neurotic, in fact the hypnotherapist can resolve physiological conditions also, for example slipped discs, trapped nerves and mysterious pains that defy conventional medical treatment.

Hypnosis can also be used to help the body heal rapidly following surgical operations or injury, I use it a lot to prepare a person for surgery to enhance the success of the operation and speed the recovery process, indeed a recent client I helped in this way reported that the surgeon and medical staff were amazed at her recovery rate. The hypnotherapist can help a subject to permanently alter his mental reactions and by doing so become more positive, fulfilled or at ease, the subject can be helped to perform better at sports, public speaking, tests and exams, and the mother to be can be helped to experience easier labour and more comfortable child birth.

Hypnosis can release such conditions as depression, migraine, panic attacks, hay fever, and allergies, eating disorders, improve self-confidence and self-esteem and many other problems, conditions and maladies far more effectively and safely than any conventional medical approach.

Since the mind runs the body and itself, a truly unlimited potential for healing and change exists and the hypnotherapist, through hypnosis, has access to this amazing power.

Further, what the hypnotherapist can do for others he can also do for himself. Right now we only need to catch a glimpse of the possibilities to spur us on and it makes no difference if you are presently sceptical or have doubts about your ability to do these things.

In all my experience as a professional hypnotherapist I have never given or implied a guarantee of any kind but in writing this book I can happily give a guarantee to provide in easy to understand language and step by step instruction all you will need to be able to heal yourself and others. To practice these self healing techniques you only need average intelligence, common sense and above all, a sense of commitment and conscientiousness.

You will only need a limited medical knowledge and must never ignore any medical advice you may have been given.

With the above qualities and some self-confidence you will be well able to achieve excellent results and amazing successes.

CAUTION when you use the knowledge and skills gained from this book to help someone it is imperative that you observe absolute confidentiality at all times. Personally I do not even discuss clients with my immediate family and if I have occasion to telephone a client I do not state who I am or what I am calling about to anyone else who may answer the phone – it could be that the client has not told anyone that they have consulted me or what they have consulted for.

ABOUT CASE HISTORIES

In this book I will relate many case histories, obviously altered to protect client confidentiality but accurate in essence. There are several good reasons for sharing these case histories. They will help you understand the workings of the mind and are used to emphasise the point being made in the teachings.

Case histories are valuable in helping you to put the knowledge gained from this book into practice.

If you have ever fancied yourself as a detective like Sherlock Holmes you will derive much satisfaction from case histories because the twists and turns and unexpected found in cases of the mind will provide a great deal of intellectual stimulation. This is even truer when conducting your own analytical work

THE PRINCIPLES OF THE MIND

Before you are in a good position to help yourself and others it is essential to understand how the mind works, a good understanding will make it easier to know what you are doing and why you are doing it.

You will also have a better understanding of why you have a particular problem, condition or issue which will help you in deciding the best likely approach to reaching a resolution.

This is certainly not a waste of time and in fact I believe you will find it interesting and fascinating in its own right.

To practice self-hypnosis it is only necessary to consider the mind as simply consisting of the conscious and subconscious parts.

THE CONSCIOUS MIND

Out of curiosity I once attended a lecture given by an eminent psychiatrist, he began by stating that we only use 10% of our brain. At risk of upsetting him and the audience I jumped up and asked what do we do with the other 27%. What the psychiatrist meant was that the conscious mind takes up only about 10% of the brain, the remaining 90% being the subconscious.

When you consider what can be done with that 10% conscious mind you begin to get an idea of what the 90% subconscious is capable of.

It is a fact that the conscious mind can only hold one thought at a time, if we attempt to hold a more the one new simply replaces the other. This is a useful trait, imagine you have knocked your ankle and it hurts and you focus on it, if you make yourself think of something else, preferably something pleasant, your conscious mind cannot focus on the ankle therefore you will not be aware of the pain.

The conscious could be described as a `part-time` mind, working when we are awake and shutting down when we are asleep, it also partly shuts down when we go on `automatic pilot` as we often do when driving long distances, watching television, reading, carrying out repetitive functions and, I suspect, when doing all this typing. A partial shut-down also occurs in times of daydreaming, `away with the fairies`, stress, anxiety and emotional or dangerous experiences. Quite often we are surprised to realise what we have done or achieved during this partial shut-down or automatic state and in extreme cases of danger we may not even remember what we did.

When fully awake the conscious mind is discriminating, selective, rational, objective and decisive. It is the analytical part of the human mind, the part which holds our conscious thought, chooses actions and takes information from around us and intellectually analyses it. While doing these things the conscious is assisted by the subconscious using memories of past experiences which were similar or connected to the current situation.

If the subconscious has a memory that calls for specific action or reaction it will normally succeed in directing the action or reaction to the present situation. In other words a past experience memory will suggest action or reaction to the current situation being intellectualised by the conscious mind, sometimes overriding the conscious mind by taking over where the situation demands, this is because the conscious mind is relatively slow compared to the speed of thought processes of the subconscious.

Perhaps surprisingly the conscious mind has virtually no memory capacity. In everyday routine activities, the conscious relies on the subconscious to provide memories of previously stored information to assist us with the current situation.

The ability to retrieve information from the subconscious is called *recall*, and unlike memory which is perfect, the ability to recall varies widely within individuals.

When appropriate the subconscious can spontaneously project the memory of previously stored thoughts and ideas into the conscious mind. This faculty is known as *inspiration*. In the inspirational experience we may suddenly come upon an amazing solution to a problem – a `eureka` moment. Occasionally ideas and thought will come to the conscious mind seemingly out of context with the present, for instance, we may have been talking about a person or place and could not remember the name then hours later when we are doing something else the name suddenly pops up.

One very useful aspect of this inspirational faculty is that we can use it to analyse and examine the mind itself, bringing about some self-revelation. This is also the mechanism that brings about the release of subconscious anxiety during analysis in hypnotherapy by returning the memory of an original negative experience (the causal event) that caused the anxiety.

This presents the conscious mind with the opportunity to resolve the negative effects of the experience through re-evaluation and intellectualisation. The recall of such repressed memories is known as an *abreaction*. The release of the anxiety or problem through the abreaction is known as the *catharsis* or healing.

A feature of the conscious mind is that we know what it is thinking; therefore the conscious mind is us. One thing the conscious mind can do for us that the subconscious cannot do very well is to deal with an original situation with creative imagination in a rational and intellectual way.

In its thinking the subconscious is only the total sum of all our past experiences that have passed through the conscious mind and have become an accepted programme in the subconscious, whether vetted or not by the conscious mind.

Unless seriously distracted by external events the conscious mind is continually chattering or talking to itself, this is a natural function and is part of its intellectualising and analytical process.

Occasionally with some people this internal self-chatting will be vocalised and where this becomes more habitual the subconscious will join in, given sufficient subconscious anxiety vocalising self-chatting can become more habitual and pronounced and can then be considered as neurotic behaviour.

Under some extreme circumstances the subconscious may take over this self-communication as if the subconscious is dealing with a problem by producing or imagining a `second person` to talk to. This secondary person is never consciously `invented`, it just becomes taken for granted that the `second person` exists. This secondary person will share his views and encourage him to talk to it more and more, ultimately leading to psychotic withdrawal.

THE SUBCONSCIOUS MIND

Way back in time of our evolution the subconscious was the only mind we had, slowly as our evolution progressed the intelligent conscious mind was developed to assist the subconscious. During this process, using a commercial company as a metaphor, it is as though the subconscious appointed our conscious as the managing director while retaining the position of chairman and holding 90% of the shares.

The subconscious has no actual intelligence and that is why the conscious mind evolved to give us this additional resource. The subconscious is our programme; it runs the entire body as well as our spontaneous mental reactions and inclinations. It is wholly animalistic, having no regard for moral right or wrong, it depends on our conscious mind to make such judgements. The subconscious works relentlessly to its programme.

The subconscious works full time, every moment of every day, even during sleep the subconscious continues to direct the processes of digestion, repair and maintenance of the body and carries out thousands of functions simultaneously. Unlike the conscious mind the subconscious can process information at supersonic speed and is able to pick up and accept information and facts about what is going on around us as *flashed* messages too brief and fast for our conscious mind to be aware of.

These `flashed` messages are referred to as **subliminal** and can become instantly accepted by the subconscious without the benefit of analysis or intellectualisation through the conscious mind. This is the reason why subliminal therapy recordings can work and help people who use them even though the volume is turned down so that the recording is inaudible.

In the USA an experiment was conducted where near the end of a movie an advertisement for popcorn was very briefly flashed on the screen, too fast to be registered by the conscious mind. As a result of this the sales of popcorn immediately rose by eight hundred percent. This sort of advertising is now illegal.

The ability of the subconscious to respond to subliminal messages is a vital part of our self-preservation, picking up on body language or sensing that something is wrong or not as it should be. Some people are highly developed in this way, often referred to as having a good sixth sense; it also gives rise to what we commonly call gut feelings or instinct.

Although it lacks in intelligence the subconscious is brilliantly clever as it remembers everything that we have seen, heard, felt or experienced since before our actual birth and has constant access to all this information. The subconscious memory is perfect and during therapy I have been able to help a client recall what was said by his parents before he was actually born and in many instances I have had clients accurately describe the events, feelings and sounds experienced during the birth process which have later been verified as true and accurate. *You will learn how to do this later in the book, it can often be the original cause of the problems a client comes to you with.*

This ability of the subconscious to remember everything and forget nothing often proves useful when helping a person succeed in exams and such because we know that the subconscious remembers everything the person has studied towards the exam and it is only nerves or lack of confidence that prevents them from recalling the information. In hypnosis we can ask the subconscious to ensure the person does recall whatever information he needs to answer the examination questions.

We have no conscious knowledge of the thought processes of the subconscious, we only experience the results of it, however, we do get a brief glimpse of the workings of the subconscious through dreams.

The subconscious is very reluctant to use words because language is the product of our conscious mind. The subconscious works almost entirely in pictures (this point should be well remembered because in inducing self-hypnosis and hypnosis in others it is wise to use words in such a way as to lead the subconscious to create pictures or an image of whatever it is you need it to think about).

During sleep, when the intelligent conscious mind is inactive, ideas and thoughts are manifested in dreams and can be depicted as distorted images and bizarre sequences. The subconscious will suddenly change scenes in a totally illogical way or produce ideas completely out of context; we can even 'see' ourselves doing miraculous things like breathing under water or flying around the world like superman.

Dr. Frank W. Lea, DD,
Dip.NLP(Master Practitioner), RPHH, APHP

ANOTHER PERSPECTIVE ON THE SUBCONSCIOUS

The subconscious can be regarded as the 'real us' with its own thoughts, feelings and reactions, this is not a case of split personality, it is the way it is meant to be. Fortunately for us it is not only the natural evolutionary way it is meant to be it is also an amazingly wonderful circumstance.

Above all else, if you want the subconscious to co-operate with you when helping yourself you must respect it and treat it in a polite and friendly manner as you would a really good friend. If you think of the human body as being a ship the conscious mind would be the captain and the subconscious the officers and crew. Neither the ship nor the captain could function effectively without the full support of the officers and crew.

Never assume the subconscious will automatically carry out a request, for instance in a normal human interaction a husband might ask his wife "can you make a cup of coffee?" and the wife would usually respond by going off to make the coffee. However, if you were to ask the subconscious "can you make a cup of coffee" it would simply answer "yes", not bothering to assume you actually want it to go and make one.

Despite its phenomenal power and capability, talking to the subconscious during therapy is rather like talking to a four year old child or someone like Doctor Spok in the popular Star Trek movies.

When working with the subconscious you must attend to detail, you must be realistic in what you ask; sometimes you will need to negotiate with it to convince the subconscious that what you are asking is realistic. Most of the time negotiating with the subconscious is a question and answer process where you receive simple yes or no answers, therefore you need to give some thought to the questions in order to eventually elicit the information required.

The subconscious will not accept suggestions or requests that are in direct conflict with your morals and beliefs.

At times the subconscious has accepted some suggestions but is unable to act upon them because of some earlier or more powerful concept, for instance if you were to keep repeating a poorly phrased suggestion like "you do not smoke" this would not help you to become a non-smoker, rather it would cause anxiety because the subconscious knows you smoke and will not accept that you do not. It is far better to say "I have now become a healthy, happy non-smoker" – this would easily be accepted by the subconscious.

THE SUBCONSCIOUS MIND'S ACCEPTANCE OF FACTS

A function of the subconscious mind is to accept facts, it stores all information it receives whether that information has been accepted as fact by the conscious mind or it has passed directly to the subconscious without being intellectualised by the conscious mind.

This means that no matter how unrealistic or bizarre a concept is, once it has been accepted by the subconscious it will run its programme as if the information were fact.

The acquired belief will remain permanently in the subconscious and will have an effect directly proportionate to the perceived importance of the accepted information. As a result, in circumstances where the subconscious is required to run the programme again it will do so using the stored information as though it were reality. In other words where similar events occur they are added to the original stored information and treated as fact. This is the basis for panic attacks, phobias and unrealistic reactions and attitudes, this process is also the foundation of our beliefs, values, convictions, prejudices and inclinations.

The same process governs our choice of friends, partners, the way we dress, colours and all other areas of selection. This principle of the subconscious mind accepting all information it receives as fact is of vital importance to the therapist, mostly because it is the basis for persistent irrational behaviour. Mostly the conscious mind protects us by vetting and intellectualising information before it is passed to the subconscious and so causing it to be stored as non-actionable information. It is the information that is accepted by the subconscious without passing through this vetting process that is the basis of problems and conditions mentioned above.

The intelligent reasoning of the conscious mind can in certain circumstanced be bypassed, for example in the stage hypnotist where a greater willingness to accept suggestions exists. Occasionally the conscious mind misses information or sees no reason to reject it; this is true particularly in times of stressful, dangerous or traumatic circumstances or when the conscious mind is distracted by some other event or task. In these situations the information goes directly to the subconscious and is accepted as fact.

Once the information is stored in the subconscious it becomes part of its programme and will come into play as part of the *normal* reactions of the person. When un-vetted information passes to the subconscious it will only resist accepting it when the information clashes with previously accepted but incompatible inputs.

This intellectual bypassing is used by stage hypnotists where they convince their subjects that they are cold or hot, drunk or are Elvis and all the other things stage hypnotists get people to do.

For the purpose of healing yourself this function of the subconscious can be utilised to help you change unwanted beliefs or reactions to desired ones, usually by the process of suggestion therapy.

MIND MODEL OF A REPRESSION

Except for our reflex physical reactions, all information is passed to the mind through our senses of sight, sound, touch, smell and taste (known as the Gestalts in NLP). Even though some people doubt its presence, telepathy does exist and could perhaps be described as a sixth sense.

The first consideration for the conscious mind is the reaction and intellectual response to input, simultaneously the reaction is passed to the subconscious for storage in memory. This stored memory of the event and the reaction to it will then be available to be used with any future experiences of a similar nature. Where the experience is registered as being threatening in some way this will automatically trigger an alarm whenever a similar experience occurs in the future.

When a person is in the normal awakened state, not in hypnosis, the conscious mind receives information and decides on a reaction to it, the information is then passed to the subconscious via the memory bank and. If the event is considered dangerous or traumatic in some way an alarm bell will be attached to the stored memory which may be repressed by the subconscious. The repressed alarm bell is constantly ringing and once activated will produce a symptom (this could be a phobia, panic attacks, obsessive behaviour or one of any number of similar reactions or conditions).

With a person in hypnosis the barrier between the conscious and subconscious is opened allowing for better retrieval of memory and access to repressed memories.

In hypnosis, when the repressed memory is retrieved the conscious mind is able to re-evaluate the event and then pass the re-evaluated memory, now without alarm bells attached to it back to the subconscious, following this there is now no longer a need for the symptom. The symptom is now permanently gone.

The subconscious has a great deal of functions to perform and many of those simultaneously, it more factual and specific than the conscious mind and it does not respond to indecisive language such s `possibly`, `maybe`, `usually`, `if` and `rather` and similar terms. The subconscious will listen to and understand such terms but they are not the natural way of subconscious thinking and it will not use them in its responses. Importantly the use of the word don't should be avoided at all times. Practice changing your thoughts from "I don't want................", to "I do want..............". For example instead of saying "I don`t want to be a smoker" you could say "I want to be a non-smoker".

The subconscious will not be inclined to repeat whatever it says; therefore you will need to develop a special way of thinking and using a slightly different language. You will often need to think rather like a detective, and this can be a most satisfying and exciting aspect.

These special ways of thinking and speaking are easy to develop and since the subconscious mind is responding in words (or causing ideo motor responses that represent words) it is essential that you are able to detect what is missing from the subconscious responses. Note that the subconscious speaking is not the same as its thinking, which it does in pictures and images. For instance, if the subconscious is asked what happened to cause the problem you have it will respond by passing the memory of the experience as a picture or movie rather than in words in the way we would consciously describe an event.

What would be missing from the words of the subconscious is the *benefits* of the problem the client has and *why the problem is there*. When asked for an explanation the subconscious might reply by saying "because it reduces the risk of the repressed experience being repeated by being more cautious".

When asking the subconscious questions care must be taken. In normal conversation, say you wanted to borrow something from a neighbour, there would be a discussion on the lines of "is it OK"?, "are you sure it is not inconvenient"?, with the neighbour giving assurances that it is fine, no problem, etc. An attempt to hold this kind of conversation with the subconscious will fail; the subconscious will not indulge in social or diplomatic dialogue. Exaggerated terms must also be avoided when speaking to the subconscious; such phrases as "I never felt so insulted in my life" may be acceptable in normal conversation but would have little or no effect on the subconscious.

Listen to yourself and others in normal conversation and if you notice that you use repetitive and exaggerated terms practice avoiding them and develop better and more positive attitudes. When I first began practicing hypnotherapy it took a while and much conscious concentration to get in the habit of not using the word `don't`, it called for a completely different way of phrasing things and actually changed my way of thinking to a more positive one.

It only takes a little thought and practice to develop this `new` way of communication and it will soon become natural to you. This new way of communication will have enormous benefits because you will be talking to your subconscious in a language that is fully understood by it.

SUMMARY

Some may think the foregoing is a waste of time and do I really need to know this.

The truth is yes, you do need to know this, and it will prove invaluable when helping yourself and others.

Most hypnotherapy courses are run as training seminars attended in person by students and most get straight down to the parts students get excited about – how to induce hypnosis and conduct therapy. Students then go away after one or two days of training and begin to practice hypnotherapy – I guarantee that 99% of them will fail as therapists unless they have a good understanding of how the mind works.

THE SUBCONSCIOUS AND NEUROTIC CONDITIONS

Considering that the subconscious is our best and most loyal friend whose only concern is our wellbeing it may seem curious that the subconscious can permit a neurotic condition to develop and persist. If by returning the memory of the event that caused the condition to the conscious mind the neurotic symptom can be easily released why is it that the subconscious does not just do that instead of allowing the neurotic condition to exist?.

Also, if the release is such a simple process why does the clever subconscious not realise the benefit of releasing the condition or even, as it does on occasion, resist the release?

There are, of course, answers to these questions but there is no single reason, the answers lie in a whole mix of subconscious perceptions and must be looked at collectively.

We must remember that a vital role of the subconscious is to keep the conscious mind as free as possible from having to deal with routine matters and also from possible distraction from itself.

The subconscious anxiety would in itself be a distraction to the conscious mind in a way similar to someone we know is very worried or upset but who refuses to tell us why or anything about what has upset or worried them. While such a person may be keeping things to themselves for an intellectual reason the subconscious is not.

This is one answer to the questions; the subconscious is not intellectually capable of understanding the benefits of releasing a suppressed memory. Also, significantly and importantly, in the same way a clock keeps time but is not aware of time the subconscious does not consider the causal event to be in the past but rather it is still happening now, today. *This is very important to remember because it will have a significant bearing when releasing repressions through abreactions.*

Example:- a female client who suffered a great deal with pre-menstrual tension recalled, during abreaction that she had her first period unexpectedly when in class at school. Her classmate noticed and made loud remarks about the fact she was bleeding and her teacher accused her of being careless and stupid.

During abreaction of this suppressed memory, rather than the client reporting that she had an unexpected period in class and was told off and embarrassed by the teacher the abreaction progressed as follows: "I can see myself in class and my tummy is hurting. I`m wondering if I`m going to be sick and need to go to the toilet. Now my classmate is pointing out the blood and telling teacher. The teacher is telling me I`m careless and stupid. All the others in the class are looking at me and some are laughing. I feel very embarrassed and frightened".

Throughout this abreaction the client was crying and I was mopping up the tears with a tissue – this when the client was now 35 years old.

This then explains that the subconscious does not see the release of a suppressed memory as the release of its anxiety, more it sees that it is returning to the event which is still happening. In this way of thinking the subconscious also regards the symptoms suffered by the client as a logical result of the event. That is A happened to cause the anxiety; therefore B is only naturally to be expected. The subconscious also regards the conscious mind as another person. This is borne out by the fact that when I have engaged in a conversation with a client`s subconscious it has discussed the client in the third person, saying things like "she does this" or "she is that". Incidentally during this exchange the client is listening in yet does not interrupt or come out of hypnosis – this seems really weird when you first do this kind of thing as a therapist.

The symptoms suffered by the conscious mind are regarded by the subconscious mind as happening to another person in a similar way to that in which a friend may be telling you he has a terrible cough and you say well, if you persist in smoking what do you expect.

To summarise, the subconscious attitude to release of anxiety through recall and abreaction is as if it is thinking "I have this experience and I do not want to look at it, the symptoms of my anxiety are being suffered by someone else and I do not want to upset him further so I can see no benefit in looking at the experience therefore I will not do it. This produces the resistance to recall that can sometimes be encountered.

Of course, fortunately there are ways to overcome this resistance and they will be clearly explained in a later chapter.

REPRESSIONS AND FAULTY PROGRAMMING

A neurotic condition may have its origins in, and arise from, any of three situations. These may be referred to as the *External* event group, the *Internal* event group, and the *Faulty programming* group. This third group however does not have to have any emotional content, nor need it be repressed to produce neurotic effects.

The symptoms of a neurotic condition can also be classified into three distinctive types. Namely: the Direct, Indirect and Contrived types. The symptom itself may be reflected in any of three ways: Physiologically, Psychologically or Behavioral.

In practice, the groups, their symptom types and reflective methods, are often overlapped, intertwined and become compounded and contorted by subsequent experiences. However, the value of regarding them in groups, symptom types and reflections, is that not only does it expand the understanding of them, but most importantly, indicates the treatment method required for them.

THE THREE ORIGINS OF NEUROTIC CONDITIONS

GROUP ONE: THE EXTERNAL EVENT REPRESSED

This is a very common cause of neurotic symptoms, and the one most referred to in this book. Put simply, to the subconscious mind, an external event takes place in which the person finds, or perceives himself, to be the 'victim' of, such as suffering an embarrassment. Alternatively, an assault, nearly drowning, witnessing a tragedy or being injured are experienced and become repressed.

At times this group can be compounded through experiencing similar events, such as a child victim of recurring parental cruelty. In such a case, just as a wall is constructed with many bricks, one experience builds onto others. In treatment, where this compounding effect has taken place, a broader resolution must be undertaken. The whole 'wall' must be removed, as if a single entity.

GROUP TWO: THE INTERNAL EVENT REPRESSED

This basically occurs as the consequence of the subconscious *itself* arriving at some erroneous but awful conclusion to some concept. The subconscious, then becoming alarmed by that conclusion, represses it to prevent the conscious mind becoming aware of it, and subsequently becoming equally upset. The Oedipus and Electra complexes are excellent examples of this and they are the most common causes of sexual problems, inclinations and sexuality issues. Internal repressions can, and often do, arise during unconsciousness, sleep, delirium, and drug induced mind- altered states.

The greatest difference between the internal and the external events being repressed is that internally constructed repressions are not released through abreaction. This is because such conclusions have not passed through the conscious mind and therefore cannot be brought back to it in a way that brings a catharsis.

Instead they must be resolved where they are, by an explanation of them to the subconscious by the therapist. The catharsis then takes the form of bringing a new realisation to the subconscious, borne of logic and intellectual reasoning. Conducted properly, the benefit of this release is equal to that of the abreaction experience.

Of all three groups of neurotic origins, the internal event repression is the least understood, or even realised to exist by many clients and hypnotherapist alike. Yet, since it can cause such deterioration in the quality of life, even causing sudden death, its importance cannot be over stressed.

GROUP THREE: FAULTY PROGRAMMING

Although this does not necessarily produce a repression as such, it is similar in that the subject has not consciously realised it occurred. To the open-minded, faulty programming will have its catharsis in self-revelation, brought about by the procedure similar to that used in resolving the internal event.

A simple example is the overweight subject, who habitually eats everything put on his plate. When he is brought to realise that he was programmed when a child, by his parents, to eat everything put on his plate, he realises that he no longer has to. That is, a change is brought about by the revelation of the programming, and unwanted food can now be left.

SYMPTOM TYPES

SYMPTOM TYPE ONE: THE DIRECT SYMPTOM

These are the symptoms directly connected to a repression, and normally in an obvious way. For example: the victim of a car accident who then finds himself intimidated by vehicles, or the drowning person suffering aquaphobia (fear of water). Less obvious, but nevertheless directly connected symptom examples include the person, once a victim of child abuse by cruel parents who, despite all his values and intentions, now discovers that he has developed such tendencies himself; or the client who reports that he is repulsed by the smell of chocolate, but can give no reason why he should be, and then during analysis, recalls being badly beaten for stealing some as a child. Since the direct symptom is a positive lead to a repression, it is usually the most responsive to analysis.

SYMPTOM TYPE TWO: THE INDIRECT SYMPTOM

Given the lack of intelligence in the subconscious, the anxiety caused by the repression is often externalised and focused onto some object or situation - this is a common origin of phobias, which, though difficult to connect to the repression becomes revealed and released during analysis. Alternatively, some mysterious illness may be brought on.

Partly in conjunction with the conscious mind, an explanation of, or some connection with the repression, is needed to account for the anxiety of the subconscious. This causes the subconscious to look for 'a culprit' and focus on that, let us say, a, in a similar way to when we are feeling unwell we seek to know 'why'? We need to know what it is that makes us feel as we do, and we need to identify a reason in order that we may take some action to help ourselves.

In just the same way the subconscious, unable to prevent projecting its anxiety into the conscious mind, will cause the conscious mind to seek to identity the cause of that anxiety, say the spider. However in doing so, the subconscious will subsequently be reminded of its anxiety whenever a spider is seen and will be made to react to the consciously but erroneously identified cause, with each new exposure to a spider, which is seen as the cause of the anxiety.

As a result the victim will seek to help himself further by avoiding the reminding situation or object. By its very nature, this symptom type may produce an abreaction that comes as a total surprise to the client, who may view it as unbelievable, or impossible. Such can be the surprise, that he may experience amazement or significant emotion, with the revelation of the experience that has been repressed. Such symptoms reflect the need for a broad analysis approach, and normally respond well to it.

SYMPTOM TYPE THREE: THE CONTRIVED SYMPTOM

This is rather a version of the indirect symptom, but is separate and different to it. These symptoms are primarily consciously constructed in response to a repression. Just as the person feeling unwell, may consciously decides to take an aspirin to make himself feel better, the contrived symptom is a consciously produced 'resolution' to a repression.

To illustrate the situation I present the following examples: "I feel vaguely uneasy so I will become a psychiatric nurse, or hypnotherapist, and distract myself by helping others worse off than myself." "Because I lack confidence, I will deliberately make myself appear over confident." "I had a terrible childhood so my children will have the best upbringing possible." Or, conversely, "I feel miserable, so I will upset others which in turn will make me feel better."

With the release of the repression producing the contrived symptom, the subject may find his occupation either less rewarding, and consequently change it, or become free to become far better at it. The over indulgent parent will normally become an even better parent, through taking a more balanced view, and the pretended confidence, will become genuine. Those who deliberately upset others will almost never seek such a release, because the others, not himself, are perceived as the sufferers. To him it's their problem, not his.

An example of this latter case is the householder who deliberately plays loud music, or has his television set on too loudly. When his neighbour, having suffered greatly, politely asks him to turn the sound down, he responds aggressively calling his neighbour a complainer, and the one who is being totally unreasonable.

THE REFLECTIVE REPRESSION SYMPTOMS

BODILY SYMPTOMS

In this, the effect of the repression shows in or on the body, apparently leaving the mind unaffected. In the 'in body' type; the symptoms can include varieties of stomach and digestive tract conditions, mysterious pains, weight problems, body malfunctions, arthritis and many others.

Where the neurotic symptom is 'on the body', a condition will exist that is usually easily medically identifiable, and be well-known of, but too often it will be 'strangely' unresponsive to medication. In the 'on body' symptom reflection, any identifiable infection that occurs will normally have arisen subsequent to the appearance of the condition, rather than the infection being the originating cause of it.

Many such 'on body' symptoms occur, but among the more common are eczema (or dermatitis) persistent rashes, psoriasis, dry skin, blushing, acne, and a tendency to look worried or miserable. By their nature, bodily reflected symptoms are not often the reason for a client presenting themselves to a hypnotherapist, for the conscious connection between the condition and the mind is rarely apparent. A notable exception to this however, is the irritable bowel symptom. Symptoms of this type may be referred to as physiologically reflected symptoms.

MENTALLY EXPERIENCED SYMPTOMS

In this second group, we have the suffering in the mind itself as the reflection of the repression. In this reflection most of all, the victim will be aware that something is psychologically wrong with him. Logically, as a result, they form the majority of those seeking the hypnotherapist's assistance. Examples of such symptoms include: depression, anxiety, panic attacks, stress, concentration lack, inner anger, inferiority feelings and timidity. These and similar conditions, can be regarded as psychologically reflected symptoms.

SECONDARY EXPERIENCE

It is a good idea to ask a client what significant event has taken place in the previous two years preceding the onset of the presenting condition or symptoms, thought any such event in itself could be misleading. It may only have served as the *key* to activate the original repression. In other words this event is simply a reminder of the original causal event - a secondary experience.

In such cases, the secondary experience is often taken by the client to be the actual cause of their malaise, resulting in the client assuming that event should be regarded as the sole object to which treatment should be directed. Frequently however, that event from the more recent past will be found not to be the real originating matter to be sought out and resolved.

A further possibility in the delayed appearance of a symptom must also be considered, and that is that that mind part, or zone containing the repression, may naturally lie dormant, serving some highly specialised function or duty, and subsequently almost never be called upon to function.

When it is re-activated, even by some relatively simple incident, it could then trigger a symptom from the original repression contained there. Conversely it could be that the vital importance of that zone of repression for other functions is such that fully repressing the original experiences becomes of secondary importance to the mind's programme having to have access or use of the zone, for those other functions. If this is the case, then it is this choice of priority that causes the repression to produce a symptom.

Lastly, in this list of possibilities, is the fact that most of the mind is unused, illustrated by our continued ability to retain a constant flow of new information, so it is at least possible that vital functions of the repression zones may be taken up by previously unemployed mind parts. If this relocation of duty area were to happen, then a symptom of the repression may never occur. For instance, it is this relocation factor at work, in those recovering from strokes and other disabilities.

Although it is far from essential for the therapist to know of the internal actions taking place in the mind, it nevertheless helps in the general understanding of the therapy to have some concept. So too does it go some way to answer why the 'link-and-connect', 'link-and-connect' suggestion, given in analysis, can have such powerful beneficial effects.

A CASE HISTORY EXAMPLE

In recounting this case history I will quote as accurately as I can the words spoken by myself and the client. This particular case is also a good example of how the subconscious can manifest symptoms of its anxiety that seem unrelated to the causal event, and, interestingly how more than one symptom can be manifested.

The client was a lady in her early 30's she came to me because her fear of needles, more specifically, a fear of having injections, was preventing her from having inoculations against disease and those inoculations required for foreign travel. This obviously restricted her choice of holiday destinations and both she and he husband were unhappy about this.

As we progressed through the analysis we experienced a lengthy abreaction which revealed more than one symptom of the subconscious anxiety.

It transpired that as a child aged five she was bitten by a dog and had to undergo tetanus injections which were painful and unpleasant to her.

During the abreaction she recalled returning home after the tetanus injections and standing in her bedroom, the room was dark because the curtains were drawn. Strangely enough she reported that she could `see` herself lying on the bed even though she knew she was actually standing just inside the room. She `saw` herself lying on the bed and then floating up to the ceiling, she was also crying, anxious and frightened.

During these proceedings the subconscious buried or repressed the event in order to protect her from remembering the unhappy and frightening experience. It also installed a programme that called for her to avoid such anxiety and fear in the future she would need to avoid injections. The interesting thing is that the subconscious also installed a programme that caused her to be afraid of tunnels.

Looking at this logically you could reasonable expect the lady to have had a fear of dogs but she confirmed that even immediately after being bitten by the dog she was not afraid of them.

Before bringing her out of hypnosis I rolled her sleeve up and told her I was going to give her an injection, I did this by gently touching her arm with my little finger nail (in therapy this is known as testing).

When she confirmed that she was perfectly comfortable receiving the injection I gave her a short suggestion therapy to the effect that she would have no problem with injections in the future and could now look forward to foreign travel. (This is known as future pacing in hypnotherapy and in NLP).

Upon returning to normal consciousness we discussed the revelation of the fear of tunnels and she ascertained that she felt sure she no longer had that problem. The two were connected to the same causal event and releasing one also released the other.

I have since received confirmation that she has had inoculations and has travelled in the 24 mile Channel Tunnel without problems or anxiety.

THE INDUCTION OF HYPNOSIS

(Self induction and the induction of others)

We have already discussed how many people have totally inaccurate perceptions of hypnosis and hypnotists that often make them afraid of it. The reality is that, in hypnosis, apart from feeling more relaxed, no other sensation is felt! Consequently, at least at first the subject is in for a disappointment at how ordinary they feel. Often complaining that they are not in hypnosis; or erroneously deciding that it cannot be induced in them, and in this latter case, deciding it must be because their mind is too strong. The fact is that often the more intelligent and strong minded people make the best hypnotic subjects.

Many people have watched hypnotists perform on stage or screen, and seen the hypnotised subjects carrying out actions or performing in a way that makes them appear to be taken over. These performances give a totally distorted picture of the hypnotherapist. The stage hypnotist's subjects act in the way they do because they both expect such reactions to occur and want them to. If they did not the hypnotist would be unable to make them do as they do.

ON REFERRING TO HYPNOSIS

By now it may have been noticed that when referring to a subject that has been hypnotised that I always refer to that person as *in* hypnosis, rather than *under* hypnosis. Although this is a personal point of view in reference, I prefer *in* rather than *under* because, to me, *under* suggests connotations with other experiences, such as under the influence of alcohol, drugs and the like or 'under the control of, under the thumb of, etc.! Each, to me, carries a negative implication, and perhaps suggest to the client that they will be under my control, whereas, 'in control, in charge of, in the driving seat and in good health', carry positive implications.

THE HYPNOTIC STATE

So what is hypnosis, or the hypnotic state? One might equally ask what meditation is. Hypnosis is in fact pretty much or the same as meditation. The good news is that hypnosis can achieve the same deep level of relaxation as in transcendental meditation but in a fraction of the time.

However, hypnosis is understood in its principles. In the following I express my own personal interpretations. Hypnosis is natural and occurs frequently and spontaneously in all of us. Being 'miles-away' is a light level of hypnosis, daydreaming, watching television, listening to music and physically repetitive actions can produce it. Hypnosis is considered by many as a prerequisite state to enter sleep.

In itself, hypnosis is entirely harmless, medically, physiologically and psychologically.

The hypnotised subject remains completely conscious in the hypnotic state, so too does the subject retain full control over himself, only acting in a way which is acceptable to him during the experience. The hypnotised subject will remember as much of what takes place after it as he would have in a non-hypnotic state. The subject can terminate hypnosis immediately and at his own behest, should he wish to - just as he might terminate daydreaming. In hypnosis the subject is more aware than in the conscious state; this is because as the conscious shuts down and the subconscious takes over and the level of awareness increases as a protection mechanism to ensure the safety of the person. The subject can also resist its induction If he so wishes.

Following the induction the only resultant feeling, if any, is of relaxation. However, despite hypnosis itself being entirely harmless, the inducer should be aware of some possible reactions in the subject prior to using the healing techniques following the induction. If a feeling of tension or anxiety is felt by the subject upon induction, then that reaction is not to hypnosis but to some existing hidden subconscious anxiety or tension becoming more consciously evident to him.

Such reactions arise because hypnosis reduces the subconscious's ability to suppress anxiety. When a feeling of anxiety results the subject should be encouraged to continue, for the therapeutic objective of the induction is to encourage changes (such as the release of anxiety through the return of subconsciously trapped emotions to the intelligent mind, and by the subject re-experiencing them). The subject should not be put off by these feelings, because even in feeling such reactions a draining away of them occurs.

Some further points need to be considered. Unless an experience of what is known as a 'spontaneous abreaction' or an 'instant recall' of a previous negative experience occurs, then any anxiety felt on induction will be mild and very easily coped with. Again the anxiety, if felt, will only be like some echo of an earlier negative experience, and since the subject clearly survived on that occasion the subject can easily deal with just remembering it.

In the event of a 'spontaneous abreaction' the subject may become very agitated, sometimes crying, shouting and screaming. To a novice therapist this can be quite frightening and worrying and he may wonder what to do. When a client attends for therapy the subconscious is already aware of why the client is attending and as hypnosis is achieved will sometimes spontaneously release the repressed anxiety and in so doing cause the abreaction to occur. In this event the therapist should remain calm and allow the abreaction to come to a conclusion, he should not 'wake' the client.

This same reaction can happen when inducing self-hypnosis, particularly when you are aware of what it is you want to achieve through self-hypnosis. If this does happen, and I stress it is extremely unlikely, just remain as you are with your eyes closed and let it work itself out, you will come to no harm and the result will be complete freedom forever from whatever anxiety you were intending to work on.

Spontaneous abreaction sometimes occurs during a hypnotic 'stage show' where the volunteer, unknown to him, has a repressed anxiety and the subconscious chooses to release that repression as the hypnosis state is achieved. Again, the stage hypnotist should allow the abreaction to conclude. It would be wise to then explain to the volunteer and the audience what had happened.

It should be stressed however, that any such reaction of anxiety, upon hypnotic induction, is fairly unusual. In the methods I put forward, no harm can come to the subject because only a memory and not an actual experience occurs. Should a spontaneous abreaction occur in you or anyone you are helping, you only need to remain calm and comforting, and resist any temptation to terminate it. For if you do terminate it you will have only done a part job and you or your subject will almost certainly be worse off.

The experience will last for only about a minute, and again, such initial experiences are very rare. However, in such a situation if you want to see someone amazed, delighted, grateful and enthusiastic, just wait two or three minutes more. No experience, in this highly beneficial therapeutic work, can be more satisfying to both subject and therapist than the release of a negative memory, whether that release be small or large in its quantity or make-up.

Whilst the recall will definitely be the essence of the moment, over the short-term it will become a 'neither-here-nor-there' matter for the subject. Beware too of resistance, which is the reverse of the spontaneous reaction, which will seek to 'protect' the subject from recalling the event. This is because to the subconscious the memory is an experience that is still currently happening and not some past event, consequently, the subject's subconscious may be reluctant to confront it.

However, as therapy proceeds, this reluctance will be proved unjustified, for not only are most repressions outdated by existing conditions, but are also mostly founded upon immature earlier reactions. What may appear to the subject's subconscious as some awful prospect instead turns out to be a simple but amazingly good experience, bringing with it a permanent benefit.

Strangely, at first sight, the recall of a pleasant or good memory of an experience has no diminishing effect of the quality of that memory. Indeed, I have experienced great delight in clients who have recalled long since forgotten happy experiences such as taking their first steps in life.

Forearmed by the cautioning points raised, we can proceed with the methods of inducing hypnosis by turning first to self-hypnosis. There are many ways of inducing it. Follow your selected process and then carry out the work you intend. You may not experience any changes in feelings following the induction procedure other than feeling more relaxed and peaceful but I assure you that using any of the methods given the hypnotic state will be present even if it cannot be felt. Most self-induction methods can be used to induce hypnosis in another person.

With practice, if not initially, sooner or later you will be able to detect its presence. In any case, it makes little difference whether you believe you have been successful in inducing it or not. Just try believing that the sun won't rise in the morning, and then check the sky the next day to see if it becomes light. As suggested, even if you don't feel any effect from the self induction, do the work you intended following the selected induction routine. Sooner or later you will be in for a pleasant surprise with your results.

THE LEVELS OF HYPNOSIS

Although the induction of hypnosis will vary from person to person, and of course from induction method to induction method, together with their various mind states during a given induction, broadly speaking four levels of hypnosis can be experienced. These are:

THE LIGHT TRANCE

As the first stage of hypnosis, this can usually be very quickly induced, and in one second. The hand passing method and similar 'instant' inductions given later are an example of this. In this the initial reaction of flickering eye lashes is very common, so too are the signs of changes in pallor, head drooping and appearing more relaxed. This light trance is the one people go into naturally as in the 'miles away', and daydreaming mentioned earlier.

It should be noted that the general rule of inductions is 'quickly in, quickly out and slowly in, slowly out' therefore 'instant' inductions are mostly used where the therapy session is expected to be short.

I once used an 'instant' induction with a nurse who had come with a trapped nerve in her neck. After de-induction she asked if she could use the method on her kids to keep them quiet sometimes!!

THE HYPNOTIC TRANCE

This is the hypnotic induction level that is most productive to the suggestion and analysis procedures given in this book, any of the signs of hypnosis may occur, but often the subject will not be aware that hypnosis has been induced, where, paradoxically, those entering the light trance will be more commonly aware that some change *has* occurred.

THE SOMNAMBULISTIC TRANCE

Generally speaking the subject will have the appearance of being asleep and because they are deeply relaxed physically they may respond with slow slurred speech, or indeed be reluctant to talk. Most such subjects will be aware that they are in hypnosis and experience feeling extremely and beautifully relaxed.

Since the subject may enjoy feeling as he does, therapy may become less productive with the subject less willing to be distracted from his sensations by co-operating with the Therapist. Such a situation can be likened to the one when we are sleepy and reluctant to talk to another. The induction of the somnambulistic trance normally requires an extended induction of hypnosis, perhaps best achieved through a combination of successive induction techniques.

THE CATATONIC TRANCE

This trance level is induced through an extended induction from the somnambulistic trance, and as such can require significant efforts on the part of the therapist. The subject is so deeply relaxed that, just as if soundly asleep, virtually no responses may be given. It is this level of hypnoses that the 'entertainer' used to place someone with his head on one chair and his feet on another, and then have a third person sit on their unsupported stomach.

Indeed the subject is commonly rigid, but will allow movements to take place which are physically conducted by another. This is also the trance level that has been used in thousands of surgical operations without anaesthetics. During this trance the subject will not only feel physiologically numb, but feel not pain either. In this trance state, should a surgical operation be performed, two significant benefits are also experienced; reduced bleeding and a more rapid healing process to follow. This form of surgical operations is routinely carried out by Dr. Angel in Spain; Dr. Angel has pioneered this technique for many years. It is sometimes referred to as Noisytherapy.

THE SIGNS OF HYPNOTIC INDUCTION

Obviously when conducting self-hypnosis you will not be able to watch for signs of hypnosis being achieved but this will not reduce the effectiveness of the work you do for yourself.

When inducing hypnosis in others it is useful to know what signs to look for in order to monitor the subjects` progress and judge the depth of hypnosis reached.

Probably the most common initial reaction from the client, particularly with the hand passing technique, is the temporary flickering of the client's eye lashes and the rapid eye movement which can be observed beneath the closed eyelids.

This reminds me of a case where, as a beginner, I decided to visit a well known hypnotherapist as a client in order to gain experience of how he worked. As it turned out, the therapist had me sit in a chair and proceeded with an oral induction. As my chair was alongside his he could not actually observe me very well and after a few minutes I opened my eyes to watch him dictating the induction into a tape recorder and he was completely unaware that I was not going into hypnosis. He was simply relying on me to keep my eyes closed and eventually go into hypnosis as I listened to the induction. I realised this was wrong and got up to leave, telling him he was useless and asking how he managed to keep getting clients. The point of this is to emphasise the importance of always keeping a close eye on the subject throughout the session.

In hypnosis some subjects will not shut their eyes completely, they are unaware of this. During this reaction they will be unable to see, since their eyeballs will have turned upwards.

Further indications of hypnosis are a noticeable change of facial pallor, involuntary facial expressions or involuntary limb and bodily movements, and the drooping of the subject's head.

WARNING

Where a person's head drops back significantly and is unsupported, there is a risk that in so doing he may inadvertently reduce the blood supply to his head by bringing pressure to bear on the blood vessels in his neck.

This is particularly so with those suffering from vertigo and being of a slim disposition. *Should a person adopt such a posture permanent brain damage could quickly occur.* In such situations it is wise to gently move the head forward so it drops towards the chest, it may also be prudent to gently tell the person you are about to do this before actually touching him.

When conducting self-hypnosis bear this in mind and ensure your head is well supported.

Dr. Frank W. Lea, DD,
Dip.NLP(Master Practitioner), RPHH, APHP

EXPERIENCES IN HYPNOSIS

During hypnosis some odd, strange or curious feelings may well be experienced, this will be referred to again in the section explaining the analysis procedure and elsewhere. However, listing such reactions and explaining them more specifically is called for. It should be remembered that during the process of recall, even if only a partial recall, that recall may be experienced emotionally (only), physically (only), or pictorially (only), or in any two or all three ways, and such recalls may be fleeting or more enduring.

Such recalls usually accompany the emergence of an abreaction by being subconsciously reminded of a repression by some connected train of thought.

Typically you may just feel emotional, but not know why. You may experience involuntary bodily or limb movements. You could feel light, as if you were about to float away, or as 'heavy as lead'. Similarly you may feel dizzy, spinning, tilting back or to one side, feel very small (physically) or as if you were twenty feet tall. From time to time it is possible you may feel sick (nauseous) or are about to vomit - although to my knowledge nobody has actually vomited.

Other things that may be experienced are odd visualised images or colours, mysterious pains, unexpected and apparently meaningless pictorial memories of some scene, or faces coming into view. If you are helping another person you should ask them to report any such reactions, *as* they occur, and not, say, following the session. Most will report such experiences spontaneously however in any case. This allows you to take such experiences into consideration with the topic or aspect of the therapy then being conducted.

REACTIONS TO HYPNOSIS

When it comes to treating yourself with self-hypnosis you already know that it is a perfectly natural, safe and pleasant state to be in. However for those readers who may be considering using the skills and knowledge gained from this book to help other people (and I hope that you do) it is worth considering what others may think in order to help them feel comfortable with hypnosis.

Some people are open-minded and simply accept what takes place. Probably fifty percent of people will vary from curiosity about the hypnotic state, through to those who are 'concerned', to those feeling apprehensive of the hypnotic induction. About twenty five percent will be concerned that in some way they will be treated in much the same way as a stage hypnotist fools around with his volunteers. This last twenty five percent will also include both those who are really frightened by the prospect of hypnosis, and those doubting hypnosis can be induced in them.

For those expressing curiosity, or lacking confidence in allowing themselves to be hypnotised, explaining that hypnosis is natural and similar to or the same as meditating or relaxing, can be helpful. Added to this they may be reassured by having an explanation of how they will feel. The hypnotic state feelings range from being undetectable to feeling deeply and beautifully relaxed. People should also be assured that at all times they will be fully aware, and be just as able to remember what takes place as they would if hypnosis had not been used.

Those who have watched the stage hypnotist at work can normally easily be reassured by pointing out that the stage hypnotist is an entertainer playing tricks with his volunteers to amuse his audience, while you are seeking to heal, and the two have *nothing* in common in what they seek to achieve.

As a professional therapist I usually find it effective, with gentle humour, to point out that if hypnosis was as they thought it to be clients would not come back for further sessions and I would soon be out of business. As an aside, I have had a few clients come who actually wanted to be `zonked out`, taken over` and simply told their problem no longer exists, in these cases I have given them what they wanted and expected – the desired results were then achieved.

Sometimes it may be that having watched stage hypnotist at work they are apprehensive, if this is the case more reassurance will be needed to overcome their doubts. (It reminds me of a client who had booked for stop smoking therapy, she arrived at the appointed time but said she was so afraid of hypnosis that she had stopped smoking so as to avoid having to be hypnotised).

Those who just express their fear but find it difficult to explain are probably expressing their subconscious resistance. In this case the resistance to hypnosis will need to be explained.

The approach I usually take is to point out what may be happening, and that it is their subconscious feeling apprehensive because it knows that you (the client) will find out what's upsetting it while you are relaxed, but rather than there being some 'tiger' in the mind, it's more likely to be some papier-mâché kitten, and that what frightens it, some long out of date issue, will probably be little more than a curiosity now.

I usually point out that *they* are in charge of their lives, *not* their subconscious, that their subconscious cannot resolve the matter by itself and the problem has gone on for too long in any case. A further way this type of client can be reassured, usually quite quickly, is by having them observe the induction of hypnosis in a third person, which can be particularly effective when the third person is a relative or friend. The hand passing and hand shaking method should again be employed in the exercise.

Quite often the issue can be avoided entirely by explaining that we will not need hypnosis in this case, just a bit of relaxation. I will then use a calming oral induction and proceed from there. Since hypnosis *is* a natural mind state, no harm can possibly come from inducing it, the person you are helping has a real need for its use and you are just doing your best for him or her. When the session has been completed you can then ask how the person feels, the answer will invariably be `great`, `very relaxed and feeling good` Then you can explain they have been in hypnosis and ask if they still think it is frightening – they will always express pleasure and look forward to another session.

SELF-INDUCTION METHODS

Choose a time and place where you are unlikely to be disturbed, unplug the phone then either lying comfortably in bed, or sitting back in a chair (remember to support your head), first allow yourself the chance to relax. If you can't relax much, begin anyway, for any relaxation prior to self-induction would only have got you off to a slightly better start in any case. Now, with your eyes closed, choose an exhalation of breath and mentally label it as a number ten, doing your best to imagine a number ten as you do so.

Should you find visualising the number difficult it is no real deterrent to successful induction but it should at least be attempted. Perhaps you could visualise the numbers as if on a door or a number just floating weightlessly in the air or some other personal mental visualisation will do. The better you have this visualisation the slightly more effective the induction is likely to be.

After visualising the ten, and on the next exhalation, repeat the method above but this time using the number nine. Now continue counting down in the same manner and include zero. Subsequently begin counting again as before, but start counting from nine and go down to zero again. Following that, of course, count from eight to zero, seven to zero, and so on, ending with the final column of one to zero and lastly with a zero itself

Repeat the entire exercise if you want to, but don't be surprised, if you do repeat it, to find yourself having drifted off into a pleasant sleep, with the intended work of course then left undone. Should you have the tendency to drop off to sleep during the first routine, experiment with shortening it to leave yourself sufficiently awake to use the hypnotic state.

THE GAZING TECHNIQUE

This technique for self-induction is better used sitting. Sitting comfortably, allow your gaze to fix on some object, say the small light reflecting and shining gently from some spot or surface - a flower, crystal or brass fitting, it doesn't matter what it is so long as it's not intrusive in its own right.

Gaze at it steadily; see details and properties in it that you may not previously have noticed. Think of its origins. If mineral, it had its origins in a supernova, the massive natural explosion of a star at least ten times the size of our sun. This rammed and fused elements one into another, and lit up our skies with a light greater than that from all the other stars of the night put together.

Somehow, through time, it has journeyed to become incorporated into planet earth, where it was eventually to be formed into its current shape. With all its properties it is now in your room, bathed in the light it now reflects, making it visible. Marvel at it, wonder at it. Its constituent parts are some fifteen billion years old. Now just gaze and think your thoughts of the great wonder to be found - even in something so small, or apparently insignificant.

Of course, you might just soak in the object's light or beauty. Whatever your thoughts, just gaze and become absorbed. After a minute or two, or when you just feel ready, say to yourself, (or think) "I'm going to close my eyes shortly, and when I do, I shall become deeply, deeply relaxed". Repeat this statement two or three times, and then simply close your eyes gently. Continue to reflect on your chosen object for a minute or so, and then proceed with your intended hypnotic state task.

<u>Note:</u> *Some people report that looking at a burning candle can produce excellent results. However, there is the question of safety to be considered should the subject then fall asleep.*

THE HANDS DROPPING TECHNIQUE

Sit, placing the finger tips together, holding the hands around chin height and a little forward from your face, and momentarily gaze at them. Then, when ready, repeat three times: "I'm going into hypnosis" follow the third repetition by dropping your hands into your lap and closing your eyes as you do so.

THE ARM LOWERING TECHNIQUE

Sit holding an arm straight out and above one leg. Gaze at a nail on one finger and keep gazing. As you gaze for about one minute, your arm with become heavier and begin slowly to lower. Try to make this lowering process as slow as possible. When the hand has reached, and is touching your knee, simply close your eyes. It is often effective to tell yourself beforehand that when your hand drops to your knee you will be deeply relaxed in hypnosis.

MUSCLE RELAXING TECHNIQUE

Another method with wide acclaim is 'clenching and relaxing'. In this, with your eyes closed, you systematically tour the entire body including neck, shoulder, face, chest and abdomen muscles, together with thigh, leg, foot, arm and hand muscles. Taking each part in a systematic order of your own determination, you first clench or tighten the muscle group, holding that tension momentarily while concentrating on that part. Then relax that part while feeling the relaxation as the tension releases. Again, the method can be repeated. The benefits of this method are both physical relaxation and induced self hypnosis.

A VARIATION OF MUSCLE RELAXING

Lie on your back comfortably with arms to the sides and legs out straight. Focus on the right arm and in your head say "my right arm is heavy and warm", as you say this focus on the arm and feel it getting heavy and warm, repeat the phrase three times. Move on now to the left arm and repeat "my left arm is heavy and warm" again focusing on the arm becoming heavy and warm. Follow this pattern with each leg, of course leaving those limbs already heavy and warm to remain so. Next, the neck and shoulders only leaving out the `warm` by saying "my neck and shoulders are heavy" After this go to the solar plexus repeating three times "my solar plexus is heavy and warm". Now focus on the heart and repeat "my heartbeat is calm and regular" while noticing it is calm and regular. Now go to the forehead and repeat "my forehead is cool and clear" while `feeling` the coolness on the forehead. Finally, attempt to imagine that you are looking into the vastness of the universe and space, referring to it is `it`, take a deep breath as you repeat "it breathes me", as you do that imagine that you have become a part of or at one with the universe and space and are drifting peacefully through it.

By now you will be completely relaxed and ready to do the work you want to do.

Note: If you have difficulty sleeping this is an excellent way to drift off to sleep, I defy you to go through this procedure twice – you will be fast asleep long before then.

THE FIVE TO ZERO TECHNIQUE

The method lends itself well to such experiences of childbirth, dental treatments and similar situations that do not require much intellectual contribution from the subject, and where relaxation would help. It is also particularly useful in dealing with sudden shock. The technique can be used alone or in conjunction with suggestion scripts to support them.

APPLYING THE FIVE TO ZERO TECHNIQUE

You simply need to count down from five to zero while attempting to picture the numbers as you do. Initially, the speed of counting may be as fast as is desired, but it should gradually be slowed if it is commenced at a fast rate.

Eventually you should aim for a rhythm wherein each number occurs as you exhale. The numbers should be repeated over and over again; *they,* and nothing else is important. The numbers are to be forced into the conscious mind if necessary and to become the dominant commanding point of attention. Everything else is secondary and inconsequential. This technique can quickly induce a state of relaxation and calmness.

DEEPENING SELF-INDUCTION

Whichever initial method you use, you can deepen it in the following way. Think to yourself, with your eyes remaining closed, "When I move my right hand I will be twice as relaxed as I am now". Follow this statement with a small gentle nominal movement of the right hand. Pause, then follow exactly the same procedure, continue with the right foot, to be followed by the left foot and left hand in sequence. As you proceed with these nominal movements and following the self-suggestive statement of "when I move my (bodily part) and saying (or thinking) "I will be twice as relaxed as I am now", the self induction becomes deepened progressively. This sequence can be repeated several more times.

These self-induction methods can of course be used in any combination you choose. It is better to experiment to discover what suits you best.

INDUCING HYPNOSIS IN OTHERS

<u>Note</u>: It must be stressed that when a subject has his eyes closed, the therapist should never, ever, touch the subject without him previously being informed of the intention.. I believe that in the USA a therapist may not touch a client without first obtaining permission to do so.

Also, take care never, to bump into them or accidentally knock them. Certainly never let your hand touch the client or their hair when passing it close to their eyes and face during the hand pass. Note too that a nose protrudes. If you do cause an unplanned or unannounced physical contact, even a slight one, trust in you by you by subject will be reduced, and the greater the physical contact the greater the reduction of trust will be, for they will just be waiting for the next accident.

However mistakes and misjudgments can occur, and if they do you will need to apologise and reassure them - it is rather a damage limitation exercise. However, in doing so, take care not to make too much of the incident.

THE HAND PASSING METHOD

In this method you simply hold your hand about 40cm from the subject's eyes, with palm turned towards them and then say: "Focus on my hand (perhaps indicating the life line on the palm, with the other hand) and in a moment I shall bring my hand down towards your eyes, when my hand is close to your eyes, it will glide down in front of your nose, lips and chin. As my hand glides down past your eyes and face just follow it with your eyes and they will naturally close then just allow them to remain closed".

The statement is spoken softly and unhurriedly. Next, having carried out the action, say "In a moment I shall lift up your right arm; there will be no shock or surprise and I want you to give me no help me at all, just let me do all the lifting". Then, gently, while standing to the right of the subject, take the right hand (hold it on the top near the wrist) and lift it about30 to 40cm and gently rock it from side to side, you may support the elbow with your other hand if you wish. When doing this it allows you to judge whether the clients` arm is relaxed or not, if it is, give praise "yes that is beautifully relaxed" or similar words. If the client has obviously helped raise the arm himself you need to encourage him to allow the arm to completely relax.

Continuing to repeat this gentle movement and then say softly: "In a moment, I shall count to three, and then drop your hand into your lap, and when I do, you will become twice as deeply relaxed as you are now." Next count aloud to three and on the count of three, allow the hand to fall into the subject's lap.

Repeat this process with the client's left hand. It is a good idea to repeat the exercise, on a first occasion with a subject, because it is quite likely that the subject may have concentrated more on what you have been doing, than simply allowing the induction of hypnosis to happen. Moreover, once the subject is more relaxed about what is to take place to induce hypnosis, the subject will just let it happen.

This induction is enough in itself for hypnosis to be sufficiently deep for work to commence. Flickering eye lashes and a slight change of the subject's posture or pallor are all good indications of a successful induction.

THE ORAL INDUCTION

In this method you merely talk your subject into hypnosis, and the following two examples will serve that purpose well. Please note however, no artificial voice projection should be used, just a gentle slowly paced, quiet presentation is best.

Bear in mind that the following scripts are just a guide, there is no need to learn them off by heart or to read them from the book, best to understand the basic intention of them and use your own words so that you can speak in your own natural manner.

A good idea for self-hypnosis is to record the scripts and play them back to yourself whenever you wish to enjoy the beneficial relaxation of hypnosis or to carry out some work on whatever you want to change in your life

Dr. Frank W. Lea, DD,
Dip.NLP(Master Practitioner), RPHH, APHP

THE TRANQUILITY INDUCTION

(Name) Please gently close your eyes (and just let them stay closed. *(Name)* Shortly, very shortly, you will begin to feel deeply and peacefully relaxed. And those feelings of relaxation are already beginning, and continue to bring an inner harmony to your mind. These feelings bring with them a sense of peace and tranquility, so that you feel more and more relaxed. As you continue to just relax and relax, you feel good.

As you become more and more at ease it doesn't matter if at times, you find your mind just wandering away to some pleasant thought, because your inner mind continues to listen, and enjoys the growing sense of peace, harmony and tranquility that is growing and developing within you now. *(Name)* You know those wonderful feelings that you can have when sleeping soundly, how you sometimes feel that you wish that you could just be left to doze and slumber. You remember how you felt, lazily laying on a lawn or a beach in the sun, perhaps drifting in and out of a dozing sleep, yawning and just wanting to stay where you were.

In a moment, I shall count slowly down from ten, and go all the way down to zero. As I do, you find that you relax more and more with each number I count, until, just as you've felt on those lazy occasions in the past, you feel deeply and beautifully relaxed once again. And as I count down I want you to feel yourself going down into calmness, peacefulness and tranquility.

Ten - feeling more peaceful. Nine - relaxing more and more. Eight - just keep gently listening to my voice, seven - breathing more deeply and breathing more slowly. Six – becoming calmer and calmer. Five - becoming sleepier. Four - just lazily drifting down, like a leaf drifting down from a tree. Three - becoming even more and more relaxed. Two - feeling as if you could just doze off into a deep and beautiful sleep. One - feeling calmer and more deeply relaxed and at peace. And zero – now you are totally relaxed, totally at peace, feeling tranquil and just resting. (*Clients` Name*) There is no particular feeling when you are in hypnosis, just sensations of peace and relaxation, all the organs of your body are working in perfect harmony and you are just feeling so good.

As you continue to listen, the sound of my voice will help you to relax more and more, and any sounds inside or outside will just be a sign and a signal to feel safe and secure and to relax even more. (*This latter statement helps prevent any sudden unexpected noises from causing the client to start and become `awake`)* I want you to have a thought simply drift into your mind. Just picture yourself looking into a beautiful night's sky, and there, in the distance, seeing one solitary silver blue star, one solitary star, millions and millions of miles away. As you watch that star twinkling in the vast expanse of space you are becoming more and more deeply relaxed.

You feel good, you are feeling ever more peaceful and as you do, just keep looking at that solitary star and soon, very soon, you will find you just drift into a deeply relaxing feeling of peace and tranquility.

Shortly I'm going to help you, and as you relax even more deeply, you will find that your inner mind responds and participates in a fulfilling and satisfying way that delights you, as you begin to free yourself to become your true self - all feelings and ideas that you want to have and grow to enjoy more and more.

Note: One problem which can occur with using oral induction techniques is that the therapist may not be aware of how the subject is reacting or responding to the induction. For instance the subject may have limited visualisation ability, or sometimes, may not find the method appealing enough. Despite this, many therapists continue their chosen oral induction techniques unaware of their client's reactions. Some clients may actually become 'bored' with the exercise if it is continued for too long.

Further to these points there is the question of speed of delivery; subjects vary in the timing they need to enjoy the maximum benefits from an oral induction. The following oral technique overcomes these problems, with the subject himself keeping the therapist informed of his participation and response.

THE FLOATING TECHNIQUE

Note: To enhance the effect of the script to follow, it is best to precede it with the hand passing method of induction, and follow this with the induction deepening counting technique.

Proceed slowly and leisurely: (*use the client's name whenever it fits in appropriately*).

"With your eyes remaining closed, I'd like you to begin to imagine yourself becoming lighter and lighter. Becoming lighter and lighter until, *(pause)* like a child's balloon at a fairground, you imagine yourself as if you are beginning slowly and gently to float up from the chair *(pause)* floating in the room. Say 'yes' when you are imagining yourself floating in the room". (await 'yes')

"Now just keep feeling that lovely feeling, it's just like the pictures you see of astronauts, floating weightlessly in space. Now, I want you to imagine yourself nearing the ceiling. *(pause)* Imagine putting your hand out to bounce gently off it, but finding that, without any sensation of contact, your arm just goes through it, followed by the rest of your body *(pause)* so that you find yourself weightless and in the room above. (or out through the roof if you

are in the top floor of a building) Say 'yes' when you are there."
(pause) "Yes!"

"Now feel yourself weightlessly, effortlessly, floating on up until you float out of the building and out into the air outside. say 'yes' when you are outside." *(pause)* "Yes!"

"Now see yourself gently floating/moving away. Look at the scene below.

<u>Note:</u> *At this junction make some suggestions with a few seconds apart, of what they might see. Suggest as if they were taking snapshots of the things over which they pass, and then keep helping with suggestions of town or countryside images that you would expect to see in your particular locality.*

"I want you to keep going now, until you see in the distance the facade of a large stately home in the country. Say 'yes' when you see it." *(Pause)* "Yes!"

"Now float gently towards it, and when you arrive, come down to land, very, very softly and gently, until you are standing on the large stone terrace in front of it. Say yes when you're standing on the terrace." *(Pause.* "Yes!"

"In a moment, when I ask, I want you to feel yourself walking across that stone terrace, and down the five stone steps which lead down to the big beautiful green lawn - feel the sensations of walking as you go. Now see yourself do that, and say yes when you are standing on the edge of the soft green lawn." *(Pause)* "Yes!"

"To your left is a beautifully carved stone vase full of beautiful flowers in perfect blossom and bloom. Just glance at it now and tell me what colour or colours do you most notice?" *(Pause for reply)*

"Now look to your right and tell me what colour or colours do you notice in the vase standing there?" *(Pause for reply)*

(Note the purpose of the colour questions is given in the section on analysis.)

You can now proceed with the appropriate therapy. On de-induction you can have the client return past the vases of flowers and ask what colours he now sees, the answers will give you an indication of the changes that have been brought about by the therapy.

The entire process, from hand passing to the conclusion with the vases, should take about three minutes or so. Naturally, some subjects respond better to some methods of induction, than they do to others. However, you will surprise yourself with your results - especially with a little practice.

A DEEPENING METHOD

Following the hand passing technique, a deepening of the hypnotic state can be obtained by using the counting technique.

Say to the subject: "In a moment, with your eyes remaining closed, I want you to count down from ten to zero, but in a rather special way. I want you to imagine each number in your mind before you say it out loud and then, imagine that number disappearing and being replaced by the next number". "As you call out each number you will find yourself becoming more deeply relaxed with each number called out". "Do you understand what I am asking you to do?" *Explain again if the subject does not.*

As the client calls out the numbers you are to say things like "deeper and deeper", "more and more relaxed" in between each number called.

Note: very often the client becomes so relaxed he stops calling the numbers before reaching zero – this is a sign he has now gone into hypnosis.

"Okay, then call the numbers out". When the subject says 'zero', say to him: "Now, with your eyes remaining closed, bring that zero back on to the screen of your mind and hold it there. Say yes when you have". *(Pause).* Yes!

Continue: "Now I'll count to three, click my fingers and that zero will just disappear - watch it go. One, two, three, 'click'! Has it gone?" *(Pause)* Yes! Repeat the counting to three and click your fingers again if the zero remains.

This procedure, used with a subject already in a hypnotic state, can be expected to take him into what is known as the 'somnambulistic' level of hypnosis.

DE-INDUCTION

Following, the induction of hypnosis, and any therapy that is carried out, de-induction is essential if the subject is then to return to normal activity. De-induction can be easily achieved by using the following script:

"In a moment, I'm going to ask you to return to the here and now, back to your normal conscious awakened state, and then to open your eyes. When you do so, you continue to remain calm and beautifully relaxed, but be vigilant and alert, so that you can do what you need to do, like driving and walking, and all in the way you normally would. Now, when you are ready, come back to the here and now, and then when you have, open your eyes and be fully awake please. Repeat the same message, should the subject be so enjoying the hypnotic experience that he is reluctant to come out of it.

An alternative and very commonly used method of de-induction is the counting up method. In this you simply say to your client "in a moment I will count up from one to five (or ten if you prefer) and when I get to five you will open your eyes and be fully awake in your normal everyday conscious state, able to deal with anything in a competent and confident manner. You will remain relaxed and feeling good". Following this you begin to count. One - floating back to the surface. Two – Coming up and feeling good. Three – getting closer to becoming awake. Four – ready to wake, stretch and smile, bringing all the good feelings with you. And five – eyes open. As you say 'eyes open it helps to click your fingers.

In all my work, I have never experienced any difficulty or problem with de-induction.

The way to deal with a person who is reluctant to 'wake up' is to firmly tell the client that they will not be able to experience these wonderful feelings again in the future unless they wake up now. Then command, with a click of the fingers, – wake up.

Remember, even if you just left the client in hypnosis the subconscious would soon realise the therapy was over and cause the client to wake up, alternatively the client would just fall into a normal sleep and wake from that in his own time.

It is interesting to speculate on how the mind has such very different capacities in hypnosis when compared to the non-hypnotic state. My own theory is that, and directly proportional to the degree that hypnosis exists in the subject, two main possibilities arise.

Firstly, (and there can be little doubt of this) the otherwise natural barrier between the subconscious and conscious minds is lowered or reduced.

Secondly, the mind's capacity to transmit and exchange memories, emotions, thoughts and reactions within itself is increased, either by reducing the electrical resistance to such transmissions, or because in hypnosis the mind experiences a heightened electrical discharge.

Whatever does happen hypnosis allows us, even more when worked on by another, to tap into that detailed memory of life that we all have. Added to these possibilities is the fact that the more we deliberately experience the state the better the results tend to become.

In the hypnotic state, we can even recall events occurring during sleep or unconsciousness, we can recall what was happening when we were in the womb, what our mother was feeling or saying and we can recall the entire birth process.

SELF HELP AND SELF IMPROVEMENT

Note: Prior to using this information it is a good idea to consider consulting your doctor for a medical examination. It must also be borne in mind that distressing and stressful experiences can occur with the release or recall of memories. Additionally a temporary deterioration in some people can be expected during therapy.

If as is hoped, the information in previous chapters have been presented in an easily understandable way, and as such, has helped you to grasp the essence of it.

There is, potentially at least, one individual who can benefit no less than others. That person of course is yourself, and you may have every confidence of success.

Most of the ways in which self-improvement and self-help can be rendered have been gone into previously, albeit though, in their use to help others.

Consequently, in using such methods for self-help and improvement, some variations or additional considerations are called for, and a definite programme needs to be followed especially since you are to discipline yourself.

Here is a suggested programme of self-help that you could follow, and it is recommended that you try it.

BEFORE STARTING

Before actually beginning ensure you are free to continue with your programme uninterrupted. If you have some distracting matter immediately ahead of you, or one that is currently occurring, it is best that you defer your first stage of self-preparation until the matter is behind you.

Such distractions might include moving home, or some important social, domestic, or business matter of a temporary nature. You need to be able to conduct your programme of self-improvement in an organised way, and as free from distraction and interruption as possible.

PREPARING

<u>Note:</u> If you intend to use a professional hypnotherapist for analysis, then you should proceed to do so prior to commencing the preparing stage, because at least many, if not all of your requirements may be met by it. Where further changes are sought, following the analysis, the four week preparation should still be followed, not least because the benefits of the analysis can, in some cases, continue to emerge even weeks after its completion and result in revised needs.

The same rules apply of course, should you decide upon conducting self-analysis, or where a friend or some other assistant is appointed to conduct the analysis for you. However, in this latter case, some initial delay may well be encountered whilst your selected aid reads these texts, and prepares himself for his role.

While many of the methods to be described will be effective when conducted by yourself, for yourself, others will be easier if you have the help of a friend and if this is your intention it is a good idea to share this book with the friend so you can both help each other by taking on the roles of therapist and client in turn. Also, when working on yourself it is a good idea to make yourself a recording of the appropriate script(s) listed later, the script being recorded following the recording of an oral induction and deepening script. The complete recording should be: oral induction, deepening, suggestion script, de-induction and can be listened to as often as you wish.

THE FIRST FOUR WEEKS

This is during the four weeks immediately following analysis, or where analysis is not to be undertaken.

You can set yourself off to a good start during this four -week period by practicing the induction of self-hypnosis once a day, perhaps at night just before going to sleep.

This will get you used to inducing hypnosis, and be preparing you further. Do not necessarily expect to feel hypnotised of course, for such feelings are more rare than common. Go through your chosen process and a sufficient depth of hypnosis will be there anyway.

To add value to your initial daily self-induction, and as a further idea for your preparations - one that is high on value and low on contributed effort - is for a minor point of self improvement to be incorporated. Any of the self-help techniques given will serve for this purpose, although the simplest are best, such as visualising some minor change as having already occurred, or 'blow-aways' for instance.

The enormous benefit of this initial self-improvement, providing you genuinely make that minimal effort, is that you will enjoy success, and see the potential for self-change in yourself at an early stage and before you have even properly set out on your chosen course. Success breeds success, just as confidence breeds confidence, and all positive results enhance the prospects of further positive progress. Just as in the reverse, and without deliberately doing so in the past, negative reactions and negative experiences may have made further negative reactions and experiences more likely.

This initial approach must be something so basically simple that it is easily comprehensible to you. You need to clearly envisage what it is you are concerned with, and what change you are working towards. A bad example would be to hold some vague idea of just wanting or wishing to be generally better, or hope in some vague ill-defined way that some symptom will just go. Rather than such an approach,

Alternatively you could deal with some personal mannerism that irritates others, or one that you wish you did not have. You may decide on positively enhancing some performance or action that you wish to improve, like sleeping better or simply being calmer. Again, you might use the future pacing technique to become more successful at some sport, public speaking or the like.

PLANNING

Your patient self-preparation, planning, and organising during the first four weeks will pay you handsome dividends, and are not to be seen as procrastinations, delays or deferments, but rather as essential and critical parts of your overall programme. There are many good reasons for the four week preparing stage, and could include any of the following.

You may wish to obtain some equipment, such as a new tape recorder, for instance.

You may wish to avail yourself of the advice given later on avoiding the media for a while, and some time may be needed for any benefit to be experienced.

You may have to construct and record personalised scripts for your own suggestion therapy. In addition, you will need time to motivate yourself, practice hypnosis and to consider your objectives.

In the period set aside during the preparing interval, you should decide what it is that you ultimately want to change, and how you intend to conduct the programme. In reaching your decisions a number of points are worth considering, and need careful thought to crystalise your conclusions. Such points may include some of the following.

You need to be open-minded enough to take into consideration things others have said of you, which previously you have denied or rejected, or that have even annoyed you when you heard them said of you. Maybe you have been accused of being this or that, told to cheer up, to do this or that, or to stop doing something, or have been conducting some aspect of your life that, say, a spouse has objected to. Ask yourself, do those others really have a valid point? Are they being reasonable? Be open-minded, stand back as it were and analyse it.

Then there are the questions of priorities, the purpose or objective of changes. Where there are several areas of self-change wanted remember that change may take time, and that it is best to take on one change at a time. Consequently, your overall progress in changing may take you months to achieve the result you desire or, say, in the case of giving up smoking be instant.

Another consideration is the sequence you select. For example, your initial goal may be to quit smoking to save money and improve your health etc., but if you do that first, and then go on to work at releasing a repression, you may then find that the way you begin to feel tempts you to return to the habit again.

A further consideration, perhaps competing with impatience borne of enthusiasm, is that rather like knocking a wall down, it is best to start with its weakest point, say a loose brick. As has been suggested, it can be best to begin with the less important changes first. You can not only gain practical experience by doing this, but build your self-confidence to tackle the more important changes you seek subsequently.

Think too of what such changes might mean, not only to yourself but to those around you. For instance, what if you have led a quiet life with little social contact, and have a spouse of the same disposition? If you awaken yourself to the joys and excitements of a richer, more satisfying outward going or fulfilling life, and then proceed with all the new found pleasures that attitude brings, what about your spouse if they should not be motivated to follow you in this?

It should be also borne in mind that perhaps, apart from a few of your 'edges', everyone knows you as you are and may broadly speaking wish you to remain the same. They may not share your enthusiastic determination for self-change. So too, your self-changes of mind may lead you to find existing ways, contacts or hobbies as less attractive, given your new found happier self.

Thought is needed, the weeks spent considering and crystallising your thoughts, evaluating plans, personal projects, priorities, methods and procedure before you begin, is time well spent in working to build up that enthusiastic self-commitment. You also need to arrange a regular time to be set aside, a specific time of the day when you will activate your plan, and be free to go into hypnosis, hopefully undisturbed.

You may also need to ask for advice from a loved one on the changes you need or plan. In short, the vital matter of self-improvement and change is not to be rushed or pitched into headlong. Your overriding goal is to become happier in some way, knowing that goal in itself helps clearer thinking, but there could be more than one route open to you.

If so, which is the best way forward? You might feel from your present perspective that improving yourself, say to help gain promotion, would lead to a greater income, more authority or security, but then, achieving that goal you might be asked to move by your company and therefore be forced to leave your friends behind.

Alternatively, upon reflection you might consider it worthwhile to change yourself in such a way as to make existing life more fulfilling and happier, perhaps taking the view that the simpler things in life are not only easier to cope with, but also often give greater satisfaction. The intention is not to put you off, for that would be absurd in the extreme, rather the intention is to emphasise the need for consideration.

ANALYSIS

A point of major consideration is whether or not to undergo analysis with a professional hypnotherapist and if so, with whom. You are free to contact me if you need to find a trusted therapist in your area.

Should you decide to select a family member or a friend to conduct the analysis the best approach, and often all that is needed, is to select somebody you can trust implicitly to take you through analysis (the friend you choose to share this book with as previously mentioned). It is essential to be careful whom you select because you may need to reveal highly personal aspects of yourself, and re-experience the events from your past that you were previously even unaware of.

It is not essential that you do reveal them, or even reveal what your symptom is or what it is that concerns you, as illustrated in the cases where the condition was simply referred to as *'The problem'*. However, it is better if you do feel free to be open, and then go on to be so.

Above all, once started, see the analysis through. Terminating analysis prematurely, say because you become apprehensive or begin to feel worse, is to risk leaving yourself in a deteriorated state. Remember, whatever it is that has happened to cause the symptom has happened, and realising only the memory of it cannot be worse than the original experience which you have clearly survived. Also, the original experience probably occurred when you were much younger, even when you were very young. What was so significant to you at that time may now only have little more than a curiosity value as a mature person. Remember too that the mind sees the event as being as real now as it was when it first happened, and holds it at that value. Time has done nothing to change the subconscious's perspective of it. The matter is now long overdue for resolution.

Again, an early termination of analysis brought about by feeling much better is also to be avoided. Some people do improve early, even following a single session, and then only to find that they slip back as another repression comes forward for release. If you have made good progress, who can say that no further progress can be made?

In one case that comes to mind, following session six, a lady rang to say because she felt so much better she saw no point in having any further sessions. However, she was persuaded to do so, and much to her surprise was to release two further major repressions in sessions seven and eight. She later reported that she could not believe how good she was then feeling, and enthusiastically thanked us for persuading her to continue.

Two other points should be stressed. The first is that analysis should run on a course with no less than five and no more than fourteen days between sessions. Analysis might be compared or likened to a course of antibiotics that are intended to be taken over a period of ten days. If all were to be consumed immediately, who knows what result might occur? If on the other hand, they were consumed over thirty days, little or no benefit might result, with the condition resurfacing or persisting.

The second point is also important. Each session should last approximately sixty minutes. Shorter sessions, by their very nature lead to less work being done, and longer ones may prove exhausting for the analist, you, or both. If you have nothing but time as the cost of your exercise, you should not be influenced in your attitude by this.

Should analysis fail at a first attempt, go through is again with a different assistant. Alternatively, find a good professional hypnotherapist who is using these techniques.

The time and any money you may spend is an investment in yourself that can have no proportional equal. Indeed, it could prolong your life, enhance its quality forever and make you more successful in some way, or simply help you to cope with some aspect of life infinitely better.

THE SELF ANALYSIS APPROACH

As an alternative to engaging an assistant or a Professional Practitioner, you can conduct the analysis or a variation of it by yourself. For this you will need more self-discipline, and almost certainly need to support your efforts with suggestion therapy recordings, both during self-analysis and following the release of your repressions.

In self-analysis you are essentially on your own, and as such must be aware of the fact that as it can in analysis by another, your problem, or the way you begin to feel could deteriorate. More importantly as you approach your self-induced release you could well, and should be expecting it, experience a bodily phenomenon (a physiologically felt experience).

Alternatively or additionally, a mental sensation might be experienced that could, without this caution alarm you or catch you unaware. Have no fear of it, such reactions last only a minute or so, and are signs of your approaching release and that your self-analysis is working for you!

Such sensations could include feelings that you are getting bigger or smaller. You may suddenly feel heavy or light, that some part of you is moving when you know it is not. Other sensations experienced may include emotional feelings, sudden images or a 'clicking' or 'popping' in the head. All that is happening is that, in the course of approaching the release of the repression, the normal sensations of the mind and the body are temporarily interfered with, rather like an approaching storm you might not be aware of, which may temporarily interfere with your television reception.

Apprehension may be experienced, but only because you are on your own during its brief occurrence, whereas the subject in the chair, with the therapist at his side, will mostly only be intrigued by it and even enjoy it.

Dr. Frank W. Lea, DD,
Dip.NLP(Master Practitioner), RPHH, APHP

CONDUCTING SELF ANALYSIS

Success is to be expected, for you have all the techniques necessary to bring about self improvements to help yourself to change. Take yourself into hypnosis by using your selected method, then with your problem, symptom or condition in your conscious mind, repeat and repeat:

"My mind is solving and releasing my problem, (or symptom, or condition) using my thoughts, my memory, my inspiration, my imagination, my dreams, my sixth sense, and my intelligence".

This, or a similar sequence, is to be repeated six to ten times at each self-session, while visualising the matter you wish to resolve as clearly as possible. As you repeat your sequence it is expressed using 'is' or 'is now', not will, which implies at some indefinite time later.

Following each of the above sessions a back-up or supporting session is to be conducted, say the following day, and before the first illustrated method is conducted on a subsequent occasion. The self-thought suggestions are also to be repeated six to ten times, but this time: "My mind is remembering and recalling". 'My mind is connecting and linking one thought to another, and recalling what caused my problem' (or symptom, or condition). Again against a similar visualised background.

Where visualisation is difficult, repeat the relative statements while continuing to be mentally aware of what it is you are telling your subconscious you want it to resolve. This version of analysis may take anything from a few weeks to several months to produce complete results, but keep going, even if you should miss the odd day or so, for it does bring results.

Following the release of a repression the self-analysis should be continued for a further week or so, but along slightly different lines. During each self-session repeat to the subconscious, in alternative sessions, firstly "My mind is recalling and releasing to me any other memories it has of the things that have upset my subconscious".

Secondly "My mind is pleased and delighted to recall things which once upset me and were repressed, because it makes me feel better and better each time that it does". Of course, should some other identifiable symptom still remain, the original sequences should be continued, with the second sequence being more of self check-up.

During self-analysis, and in many other cases too, the questioning, reasoning and negotiating methods can be incorporated, and often to great beneficial effect. Where you use this method any mental object can serve as the 'yes/no' indicator such as requesting the subconscious to have a green sign saying 'yes' or a red sign saying 'no' to light up in the mind.

FURTHER SELF-IMPROVEMENT METHODS

Using this method, and following the self-induction of hypnosis, you see yourself at various intervals in the course of some activity, such as being and feeling highly successful and enjoying yourself, confidently conducting the activity to a highly successful conclusion. The pictures may be only brief snatches, and the actual (if any) words can be left to one side, for they are not normally important.

Except where you want to imagine some particular words to be said that represent specific success, like someone important smiling at you enthusiastically and saying "Well done, well done" or "Fantastic" or "Brilliant" and the like at some stage or conclusion of the activity make both pictures and the good feelings as intense as possible, and make them as real as if you were *actually* experiencing the event in the way you picture it.

The concluding scene is normally the most important, for it follows a successful completion of the event, and in doing so clearly instructs your subconscious in the intention of the outcome that is desired.

So important is this visualisation and good feeling with the successful conclusion of the event, that at times it will be entirely sufficient to bring about the required positive result or outcome in a real situation, following just a single attempt with the method.

This technique can be used for many situations, in some general sense or some particular circumstance, such as when you find yourself nervous, shy, self-conscious or under some stressful pressure - like having to make a public address, being involved in some special occasion such as a wedding or some social gathering, or alternatively, feeling apprehensive over some forthcoming event, such as visiting the dentist, taking an exam, an interview or meeting some important people. In all of these it is the successful finished result, and the final satisfactory outcome that receives the intensive visualisation and good feelings.

The subconscious does not differentiate between an intense and vivid imagined event and an actual one, therefore when you intensely and vividly imagine something taking place as if it really was happening your subconscious will accept that this has actually happened and will store the memory in the same way it would store the memory of an actual event.

For example, let's imagine that you have negative feelings about speaking in public. You then visualise seeing an appreciative audience, having concluded your speech, and knowing it has gone amazingly well. You have excelled yourself; you have given a brilliant, logical, enthusiastic, free flowing speech. You have been relaxed, enjoyed it, remained calm and totally convincing; your mind has been alive and inspired. Your pacing and delivery was perfect. You are now aware that you have delivered your final words and sat down, or stood back, feeling intensely good. Look briefly at the real or imagined faces, see their enthusiastic acclaim, see them clapping, clapping and clapping whilst you feel really good, this is really happening to you, and right now! Next see, not necessarily imagining the words used, someone thanking you for your brilliant delivery, see them stumble to find words good enough to reflect their gratitude and admiration.

In an exam situation you see yourself relaxed, clear thinking (don't bother imagining questions or answers) and just feeling good because the questions are so easy, see yourself amazed, delighted and proud with your finished result, see the confirmation of your passing, again not the words, but holding the actual letter or certificate that confirms your successful achievement. Hear the examiner saying you have done well, passed etc. See his congratulatory expression.

The same principle goes for interviews or meeting important people. You know you have done exceedingly well, your hand is being shaken enthusiastically, or the facial expressions given to you by them are saying you are appreciated, admired, respected, needed. In sports see the ball rolling or flying to the exact chosen target, see that dart sinking into the board at the exact spot intended. Hear the acclaim, feel the jubilation inside yourself. In making something, particularly if while being watched, you see the object coming into shape, see it finished to perfection, feel good, calm and relaxed, see the appreciation in others and feel it in yourself as your finished product is displayed.

With these self-suggestions and a little imagination, any of a wide range of activities or events can be incorporated into the general principle. However, never visualise in the negative mode, like seeing yourself not reacting in a given way, like seeing yourself not being nervous or self-conscious. Such thoughts may well serve as reminders of what you have feared, and inadvertently, raise your awareness of such possibilities. In fact, without any use of hypnosis at all you will see some positive changes just by changing the way you think and the words you use in everyday life by avoiding thinking about what you don't want and always thinking about what you do want, change "I don't want to be nervous" to "I want to be confident" or "I am confident". Whatever you focus on your subconscious will strive to help you get and when you think about something you don't want your subconscious has to picture this in order to understand what you are thinking and therefore is focusing on that thing you don't want – better to make it focus on what you do want.

Rather than negatively seeing yourself as not being nervous or self-conscious, see yourself with these reactions absent. See yourself as being, feeling, and acting in a confident way, or enthusiastically engrossed in what you are actually successfully doing.

What happens in all of this is that you are clearly programming your mind as to how you expect the final outcome to be. You are telling your subconscious how to react, and how to conduct the affair to bring about success, and more importantly, how to make success the conclusion of the matter. The subconscious, now clearly fixed on the positive objective, will use all of its enormous resources to make that chosen outcome become a vivid reality.

Compare this positive approach to the more common negative approach and subconscious negative programming, unintentional as it may be, of "I know I will fail", "I know I shall mess it up", "I shall be embarrassed", "I am so self-conscious", (or nervous) "I dread it", "I can't do it".

SELF-SUGGESTION

In hypnosis, and set against some visualised mental picture, you repeat over and over a phrase thought out in advance. Such a phrase might be "I'm becoming more interested in what I enjoy studying, because I'm learning more and more all the time". This is repeated, not as some kind of wish, but a statement of logical fact.

Other examples include: "Every day I get better at my job, because I become more experienced", "I'm becoming more confident, because I feel more and more self-assured", "I make more and more progress, because I get more and more satisfaction from what I am doing".

This is not the same as repeating affirmations in front of a mirror as some books suggest, they are pointless unless you actually believe the affirmations to be true. The positive self-suggestions need to be clearly emphasized with strong visual images of yourself actually being what it is you are saying.

Even if you should think, in your conscious mind that such suggestions are great desires but out of context with what you believe to be the actual situation, you will soon find that in carrying out such repeated self-suggestions gradually the suggestions will take root, and bring them into reality.

BLOW-AWAYS

In blow-aways create a mental image of some unwanted situation or person while in hypnosis and holding that picture steady, take a deep breath and blow it away. This simple technique is amazingly effective and can be applied to a huge range of situations. It is also a good technique for children to use on things that are bothering or disturbing them.

PROBLEM SOLVING

The method is simple. Go into hypnosis, examine or think of the question or problem to be solved and focus in on it. Then, having brought your subconscious to concentrate on the matter, simply repeat "My mind finds a solution, my mind solves this problem for me, my mind inspires me with a marvelous idea/ solution". This principle can be used for matters in your private life, business affairs, work, or any other area.

One of the most amazing examples of it I heard about involved a hypnotherapist who wanted more clients when practicing as a hypnotherapist, he repeated to himself the instruction that his mind would arrange for him to have more clients. During the following ten days he had four new clients present themselves for analysis - a Mrs. Moor and three Mr. Moors. Coincidence! I think not, rather a slight misunderstanding by his subconscious, which had used a mass broadcasting telepathic solution. Surely it would be a fluke of immense improbability, that following the use of this method, the only clients to contact him should each be called Moor.

This illustrates the need to be precise about what you are asking for, it would, for instance not have been helpful to visualise a queue of clients at his door when in reality clients would normally contact by phone to make an appointment, therefore he would need to visualise clients doing exactly that.

CALLING-UP THE SUBCONSCIOUS

In hypnosis, you tell yourself that the subconscious is coming forward into your mind in some pictorial form or representational way. Gradually, or more commonly suddenly, a picture like some hologram will appear. It might take the form of a flower, like a beautiful red rose, or a disc of light, an apple, a bush or star. In my case it appears as a dandelion. It can help to achieve the objective if someone is with you and suggests it, and follows the suggestion with the one, two, three, 'click' technique. In the absence of an assistant you could try this yourself.

The point of this exercise is that you then have an identifiable object with which to mentally communicate, whilst being in direct communication with the subconscious itself By using clear simple questions, affording either a 'yes' or 'no' response, you can then proceed to engage in an information exchange, albeit in a restricted way, since only 'yes' or 'no' is normally the response from the subconscious in this method. A 'yes' or 'no' might well be given by say, a nodding or shaking of the symbol, just as a head might be used to express 'yes' or 'no'.

Alternatively some change in the symbol will represent the answer. It is best to use this method for the more simple matters, like saying to the subconscious symbol: "Will you agree to send me into a beautiful and deeply relaxing sleep tonight?" Given a

"Yes" answer you should find some pleasant soothing thought enters your mind, a pleasant scene or picture, perhaps a gentle stream, flower or cloud formation and shortly after, drifting off to sleep.

A similar question might be for you to have a 'sexy' or romantic dream that night, or for your mind to waken you at a certain time, or of course, for it to agree to find that elusive solution to some matter.

POSITIVE AND LOGICAL

The opposites of which are pessimism and irrationality, in the sense intended here. Most people lead their lives somewhere between each pair. Whilst pessimism can be more justifiable, and even be reasonable in certain respects, such as 'doing the Lottery' but feeling pessimistic of winning millions of pounds, irrationality can never be justified. Ironically, being over positive can have adverse effects when carried to extremes, such as pursuing an expensive lawsuit, positive that you are right and losing when proved wrong, and being as if blinded to reason.

In the sense that being positive is intended here, you are confident rather than over sure. Unlike the risks of being unduly positive in the *'so cocksure of himself'* style, logic, ultimate logic, cannot be found wanting or erroneous, because if found so it must then be considered illogical.

The point intended by this, is that in helping yourself (and unquestionably in helping others) you are dealing in logic that may conflict with beliefs, just as being positive conflicts with being pessimistic. In hypnotherapy, special mental attitudes of open-minded ways of thinking and reacting are called for to an extent which may not be so essential in other aspects of life. In working to improve yourself you need to be forearmed to deal with the unexpected conflict between belief and logic.

FURTHER CONSIDERATIONS OF LOGIC

It is illogical to argue with the subconscious, illogical to tell it what to do, especially in the direct commanding sense, but logical to question it, reason with it, and negotiate with it. It is possible to say to the subconscious that you accuse it of something, like holding a guilty secret, providing that in doing so you can justify what you say with logic.

Logic should be encouraged to enter every aspect of your life, for example when something goes wrong for you, you are entitled to feel disappointed, but anger, by itself being the sole response, serves little more than to aggravate the situation. Illogical and irrational behaviour can be seen all around us - on our roads, in arguments, and at work places.

We can be illogical even where no other person plays, a part such as Basil Fawlty snapping off a branch of a tree to thrash his car for annoying him with its mechanical failure, whilst shouting "I warned you, I warned you" in the highly popular Fawlty Towers TV comedy series for instance.

You can help yourself enjoy a greater satisfaction from life, and gain more respect from others by becoming more logical, not annoyingly so, giving the impression of being always holier than thou, for that attitude is in itself illogical, but with humour and understanding. Be aware of what you are saying, ask yourself if you are being logical in all you say? Can you justify yourself, if need be to yourself above all? It's also a good idea to remember to avoid routinely using hackneyed expressions, and use alternative expressions to present your point, or consciously and deliberately use them selectively.

As you become increasingly consciously aware of your logical ways, you will become equally aware of the illogical ways in others. You will also have improved yourself, and considerably underlined the value of the views you hold, and in what you say and do.

A favourite example of mine that further illustrates what has been said in this chapter, is that of treating a client for a loss of confidence, and is infinitely better than the suggestion approach since it is based upon undeniable logic. Following the discovery of the cause of the lost confidence and the resolution of the experience, it then comes to the point where the confidence is actually to be restored, and can be done so along the following lines.

"You were born with total confidence. Sometimes something happens to cause the subconscious to feel that, because of the experience, confidence is inappropriate and because of this, confidence is reduced or partially withdrawn. In this, the subconscious is seeking to protect us by holding us back to avoid further exposure to some imagined vulnerability. Subconscious, is that what happened?" "Yes".

"But, subconscious, that lack of self-confidence becomes visible to others who then feel free to take advantages, perhaps mock, embarrass or intimidate us, sometimes making us angry or reducing confidence further as an extension of the imagined protection. Subconscious do you agree that this is true too? "Yes". If I could offer a far better protection idea, one that really works well and solves all these problems, would you be prepared to consider accepting it?" "Yes".

"Subconscious, if instead of reducing confidence to protect, and finding that approach fails to protect, you were to restore totally all the confidence you were born with, then you would hold all the advantages. Others would respect you and no longer be able to take advantage, for you would be as confident and as assertive as any other person, and be able to actually protect yourself perfectly well and also enjoy life far more.

Subconscious, would that be a better, more attractive and fulfilling method of sound protection?" "Yes".

"Does any part of the subconscious object to accepting this wonderful method of protection?" "No". Then, subconscious, I will count to three, click my fingers and you do whatever you need to, to make that method of protection a full reality. One, two, three, 'click'." - (Actually doing this if you are using the concept on yourself).

The method works wonders because it is based on undeniable positive logic.

IN CONCLUSION

Please go back over this section but on this occasion, rather than reading it study it. Read between the lines as it were; ask yourself what is meant, rather than only what is said by it. For, if you are working on yourself by yourself, you need to be your own expert and to understand not only how, but what you are doing, especially in order to deal with the unexpected, such as experiencing a spontaneous abreaction.

Should that occur you will know what is happening and what forces are at work. Instead of being frightened and terminating it, you can see it through and deal with it, and in a knowledgeable professional way. In all of this, I do not wish you good luck, for good and bad luck cancel each other out in the long run, but rather that I wish you well.

DE-INDUCTION SCRIPT

"In a moment I'm going to ask you to come back to normal consciousness, I will count up to 5 and on the count of 5 your eyes will open and you will be fully alert and able to do whatever you need to do in a calm, confident and competent manner. 1, beginning to awaken, 2, coming up, 3, 4, getting ready to wake up feeling wonderful, and 5, eyes open, feeling great.

Further suggestion scripts are to be found later in the book and are a guide to recording your own for yourself. Because of the wide variety of possible uses, only the more common examples are covered but they will be of considerable value to understanding the basic principles of writing scripts which will enable you to make up your own.

Illogical or non-positive phrases will be inverted from the intended result. "You are not nervous or jittery" is intended as positive but will create a picture of the nervous jittery state that he sees himself in already. Consequently the suggestion may compound the condition, and have the opposite effect to the intention.

Saying "be careful!" to someone carrying an overfilled glass of water, or saying "be careful you don't spill it" carries the picture of the water being spilled in the subconscious, which would then likely result in the water being spilt. Similarly the word `don't` has no meaning to the subconscious therefore `don't do such and such` will be translated as `do it` because the subconscious will have to create an image of the thing being done in order to understand the instruction.

In other words "you are calmer and more relaxed" creates a picture of calmness whereas "you are not anxious or nervous" will create a picture of nervousness and anxiety. "You prefer good nutritious food" is far better than "you will not eat junk food".

Forgive the repetition, but to emphasise this vital principle, I say again negatively phrased suggestions, despite what is intended, actually promote negative results. A further point to be stressed again also is that all such ideas transmitted to the client which will be converted into pictures in the subconscious therefore you always need to choose words that create the desired picture with no room for misinterpretation.

In hypnosis, that picture is accepted as fact, and it then becomes the goal or aim of the subconscious to bring it into reality. Since it is not the task of the subconscious to decide if such a mental picture is in the real interest of the person as a whole, negative suggestions or pictures can be as actively accepted as positive ones.

However, the negative picture can be very useful, in that it allows some concept to be put forward in a way that doesn't 'attack' the listener, but heightens comparison with the desirable alternative such as comparing the health risks of smoking with the pleasure of not smoking thus making the pleasure more desirable. So too, suggestions should not include highly emotive words, like pain, danger, death, dying, rage, anger, violence and so on. Except in the anti smoking script for example, where such words are used to refer to other people.

Imagine, for instance, the highlight that the word 'pain' would produce in a client, fearing what she might experience during the birth of her first child in the following: "You will feel no pain as you give birth, giving birth will be pain free." Compare that statement with: "Giving birth will be easy, smooth and a pleasant, natural experience".

Which statement creates the more desirable image?

In addition to such suggestions, the client who is, say, fearing the dentist or some other event can be taught the technique of mentally counting down from five to zero repeatedly during the experience.

By using this technique significant additional relational benefits will be felt. I quote verbatim from one letter that I received, written by a lady who had considerable apprehensions at giving birth, who came to me for help.

It might interest you to know that I had a virtually pain free labour, not one panic attack during the five days in hospital and most amazingly did not have to use any of the morphine based pain killers which they wanted to give me after the caesarean operation. I am totally convinced that the relaxation techniques you taught me made a tremendous difference.

Such is the value of analysis (to uncover the cause of her fear) followed by good suggestion therapy, supported in turn by teaching her the relaxation technique.

Suggestions that the client will act out of his fundamental character will not be accepted.

As previously put forward, suggestions must either be logical, or supported by logic. The client, lacking confidence for example, may find it difficult to accept the concept of acting confidently, because he cannot accept the positive concept as being possible. However, where the suggestion is reinforced by logic it can then be accepted in its positive form

It must also be stressed again that suggestion scripts, either recorded for listening to or for reading out from, are mainly intended to 'top-up' or support earlier work that is, where either a repression has been released, or some earlier connecting experience has been recalled and dealt with. Although suggestion therapy may be used to help tide someone over some special forthcoming situation, or simply to change mental perceptions and unwanted habits, they should never be used solely as an attempted 'cure' for a neurotic symptom or problem.

It will be seen that most of the suggestion scripts have much in common, seemingly almost repetitive in content. This is because the fundamental principles themselves are basically simple and few in number. Reading through the scripts will provide the knowledge, by way of their example, that you will need to prepare your own versions. These scripts should also be varied to fit in with the differing personalities that are encountered.

Since the subconscious works at a far higher speed than the conscious mind, the speed of script delivery is secondary, although irritation may be caused, should the delivery appear rushed or hurried. Enthusiasm and emphasis in delivery helps, though they are not essential. Nonetheless, delivery should flow smoothly and in a natural way of speaking, strange and artificial ways of talking should be avoided, though a slower pace and a calming tone of voice can be used.

Since most people talk differently from the more grammatically correct way they write, the script becomes more natural if delivered in the same way as the spoken language is used. 'You will' is perfectly acceptable as 'you'll', and punctuation can be used in a way that would be unacceptable in good written language. Repetitions and shortened words are also acceptable during delivery. Dated references should be avoided, for instance in a script to raise general confidence when attending meetings part of a programme of change in overall attitude at meetings it is no use mentioning meetings to be held on specific days.

RECORDING SCRIPTS

In the recording for self-use you can incorporate your own name, such as in the third person sense, 'Harry is', 'Harry has etc., or speak as in the first person: 'I am, I have' etc.

Where a script must be repeated, it may be presented in full on the first occasion, or a second occasion where there is a time interval, and then be reduced to the more basic essential ingredients for further repetitions.

Where the scripts are recorded it is essential, particularly if intended to be used repetitively, that they should be free of distracting intrusive sounds. Having a pneumatic drill going off or a door being slammed in the middle of a recording could cause the listener some annoyance, (an annoyance that will also be subconsciously recorded and could be adversely associated with the subject of the script) in addition to it distracting the listener in subsequent replays. He will be anticipating, it and wanting to get that part of the recording over with.

The professional hypnotherapist produces good quality recordings, having rehearsed and practiced the script before making his final version. Such practice also helps to avoid producing a recording with 'clicks' on the tape, where the tape has been rewound in order to wipe out some part that was wrongly read originally. The recording of a suggestion tape that is made in two or more sittings is also to be avoided, as this could suddenly cause a distracting shift in tempo, volume or voice sound.

One further point previously touched on, but one which will benefit by repeating it with individual emphasis, is that the suggestion must in essence be realistic. Whilst immense changes can be achieved, with goals seemingly unlimited, no suggestion of obtaining the impossible will make that impossibility somehow available. The disabled man cannot instruct himself to re-grow a lost limb, though he may instruct himself to perform physically better, or to adopt a more positive attitude to his disability. We are a very long way off suggesting to somebody that they can fly to the moon, and subsequently finding them doing so.

Before closing this section, I feel drawn to return to the stage hypnotist, whose 'entertainment' is condemned by some hypnotherapists. Occasionally a hypnotherapist has a client who thinks that what they see in the stage hypnotist act is what can be expected from the therapist. I usually point out to them that one is a hypnotist and an entertainer, while the other a hypnotherapist and healer. For some people stage hypnotism gives a totally wrong impression of what hypnotherapy is, or can do. Witnesses will say: "Just look at the ridiculous antics hypnotised people can be induced into performing".

Some would-be client's for hypnotherapy watching the stage hypnotist, may be put off hypnotherapy by this, and as a consequence, lose the opportunity to avail themselves of what in many cases is their only hope for self-change. I have occasionally had a client who asks if I can make him run around like a headless chicken as he has seen on a stage show and I say yes, I can if that's what you want but it will not help resolve your problem, the point is though, if your subconscious is powerful enough to make you do that it can certainly help resolve your problem.

The fact is that hypnotherapy evolved from stage hypnotism and personally I know for sure that learning stage hypnotism increased my success and effectiveness as a hypnotherapist greatly because it gave me an even deeper understanding of how the mind works, a lot more confidence in dealing with people and I learnt new techniques of induction and ways to enable me to convince a sceptical or nervous client that hypnotherapy will help them. I particularly find that the skills of the stage hypnotise come in very useful when giving public talks and presentations which gain me many therapy clients.

EXPECT THE UNEXPECTED

People respond in hypnosis in so many different ways it would not be possible to list. While mostly people will respond in similar fashion to the examples given in this book you must always be prepared to deal with totally unexpected reactions, that is why it is so important to understand how the mind works because on many occasions you will have to think on your feet and make up responses or procedures on the spur of the moment. I quote a couple of amusing and unexpected incidents here.

A client called to arrange stop smoking therapy. He arrived, he was a big, powerful, rather intimidating businessman obviously used to having complete authority.

On his arrival he said that because I had helped his friend stop smoking I would be able to help him. "So stop me smoking" he said. I invited him to come to my consulting room but he said "I can't be bothered with that, just stop me smoking", again I tried to get him to come to the consulting room and once more he said "I don't have time, my friend said you could stop me smoking so stop me smoking". I could see this was going to be a bit of a battle so on an impulse I looked directly into his eyes and said in a very commanding voice "You no longer smoke" at the same time I clicked my fingers right by his ear. The client said "thank you very much", paid me and left. I later heard that he never smoked from that day on. Obviously his belief and expectancy was very strong and he believed that if I told him he would not smoke then he would just quit. You will not find instructions to use such a technique in any hypnotherapy course anywhere – you just have to make things up on the spur of the moment sometimes.

Another incident which obviously stemmed from inaccurate perception of hypnosis, probably due to bad media presentation of hypnosis is a good example of how powerful pre-conceived ideas can be. A client arranged a session for stop smoking therapy, it is quite common for people who book for smoking cessation to change their mind and not turn up, however, in this case the lady was polite enough to turn up at the appointed time. As I opened the door to her she said "Sorry, I don't need therapy now, I was so afraid of being hypnotised that I have quit smoking so I won't have to have a session and be hypnotised. I thanked her for being polite enough to turn up and off she went. I didn`t get paid for this one.

Life is wonderful, people are wonderful and we learn something new every day.

SUGGESTION SCRIPTS

SEQUENCE OF RECORDINGS

Although some will want to make their own therapy recordings I recommend that it is easier to purchase professionally produced therapy recordings which are available very cheaply from www. ukboard.org

I have included scripts for some common issues but if you require a script for a specific issue not covered here you only need to email me and I will happily send you one. They can also be found on the above website.

When producing a recorded suggestion script, unless hypnosis is to be induced by some other method, an oral induction must be included at the beginning. For legal purposes a warning not to listen to the recording whilst driving or doing anything that requires the listener`s full attention can be included if you intend to pass on your recording to other people. Advise the listener to sit or lie down somewhere where he is unlikely to be disturbed. The first words on the recording should be spoken very softly, so as not to disturb the listener. Recordings to be used by the general public cannot, of course include a person`s name as you would in a script used for self help therapy.

If you have the facility to record your voice over background music, find a piece of music which does not have copyright problems and lasts at least 45 minutes. A suitable background music recording is available from www.ukboard.org as is a subliminal recording to be used in therapy which greatly enhances relaxation in the client.

A longish oral induction as supplied in this book must precede the actual script or, of course you can use your own.

Scripts should be concluded with future pacing visualisation of the listener visualising experiencing his everyday life with the benefits of whatever the script was for. "Just as it is possible to see into the past it is also possible to see into the future and I want you to see yourself one week from now doing...........now see yourself one month from now doing.........even better, one year from now enjoying your new ability/freedom (as appropriate) as a natural and permanent way that you are" is a good way to guide the future pacing.

De-induction as described in previously is used, bringing the listened out with excitement at enjoying his new future free from......or with.......whatever is appropriate.

The following scripts are meant for guidance only. They need not be learnt verbatim and I suggest you adjust the wording to suit your own style of speaking and tailor the script to suit the needs and requirements of yourself or whoever you are helping. Use these scripts as a guide on wording scripts, this will help you to write a script for your own particular requirements.

HEALTH

<u>Note:</u> As with lack of energy, it is essential that the exploration of causal factors be undertaken. Certainly a visit to a doctor is essential. In the script that follows, it is the person who is receiving medical care already, the person whose resistance to infection seems low, the person with hypochondriac tendencies or someone recovering from some illness and requiring a mental tonic that is in mind. (The person with a low resistance to infection could also be recommended to try a course of primrose oil, the 'King Cure' remedy.)

In a moment (Name) I'm going to help you, I'm going to help you by showing you how easy it is, for all your natural self-healing properties to be activated. Just relax and continue to listen, as I explain this simple idea. You see (Name) you have _all_ the natural resources to enjoy good health. Your subconscious mind knows precisely what to do, and how to make you fit and well, and to keep you that way.

As I speak, all those natural forces you have are being assembled, marshalled, and called up, and because of this, are all coming into vigorous action. You are getting and feeling better with every second that passes, because the process has begun instantly, just like throwing a switch. (Name) You are now returning to perfect health, your natural defences are growing, and your immune system is developing in leaps and bounds.

It makes no difference whether you believe it or not, because the result is the same anyway. For your entire system is receiving all the help and assistance, that makes good health a natural and continuous process. Some people describe others as the picture of good health, glowing, or radiantly healthy. In such people, as if by some luck or happenstance, all that has happened is simply that all their natural good health preserving mechanisms have just been triggered into action – there's nothing more to it than that.

Such people expect to be fit and well, and their mind simply takes up that healthy concept and runs the programme in their inner minds. Such a programme is not only easy to take up and run, but actually saves the mind energy and effort because it no longer has to deal with unwanted poor health conditions.

(Name) You see it is far easier for both your mind and your body for you to **be** in good health, since as you become stronger, your resistance grows stronger too. That in turn makes you stronger still, and leads again to a further increase in your natural resistance. Leading you too, to that radiantly healthy picture I mentioned just before. (Name) Although you may not realise it, in your subconscious that picture of you as radiantly fit and well in every respect, is forming clearly.

Your subconscious is focusing in on how you are becoming, and is increasingly becoming more enthusiastic, determined and eager, to make that picture a glowing healthy reality. And so swiftly have you changed to that healthier state, that it amazes you and all those who know you. With your new found glowing health, comes the energy that health brings too. You enjoy all the pleasures with just feeling good, and feeling wonderful.

This exciting change, that has already begun, is growing and developing now. (Name) You are already feeling better, stronger, fitter, more energetic and happier, and in every way too. The process of progress is continuing, minute by minute, hour by hour, and day by day and week in and week out. Your subconscious does all this for you, leaving you to just enjoy being the healthy way you have become. In short, (Name) congratulations, and here's to your good health!

EMOTIONAL SELF CONTROL

(Name) Shortly I'm going to present you with some pleasing and constructive ideas, and all for your well-being, happiness and satisfaction. These welcome ideas take root in your subconscious, to help you to be the natural way you want to be.

(Name) For so long, in the past, you've been feeling and acting in ways that have detracted from your natural personality, and leading you to feel less fulfilled. Now, as I continue, you are realising that there is a better way of feeling and acting. A better way that brings· pleasure, satisfaction, and a far greater harmony into your life - a far more logical way of conducting yourself

(Name) You are becoming calmer, more rational and reasoned, and you find that by remaining calmer, more rational and reasoned, that you express yourself more persuasively, more agreeably, and more intelligently. That as you remain calmer and more rational, you think more quickly, more intelligently and are more able to express yourself in a logical way that commands great respect, in both yourself and in others.

In your new calm way, you can more easily see the points others wish to make, with you responding with logic and reasoned responses. You respect, like and appreciate yourself more and more, with each experience of calmness and control that you now find in yourself.

You do have a calm, reasoned approach, and in every way and to every matter. You always remain relaxed, peaceful and logical; above all, you take an immense pride and great satisfaction in your balanced judgment, relaxed attitude, and the confident manner you have, that delights you. For you do always remain logical and calm. Others, as well as yourself, admire the wonderful way that you just take everything in your stride, and the way you are able to see the amusing and funny side of things. The way you are able to take things in, and understand them more.

(Name) You become calmer, and more relaxed and in control with each and every experience of these pleasant, intelligent, logical feelings and reactions.

(Name) You are always calm, and reasoned, making your life richer, happier, and more self-fulfilling. And in all of this, (Name) you are to be congratulated.

ACHIEVEMENT / MOTIVATION

(Name) As I continue to talk to you, a wonderful feeling of determination is beginning to develop inside you. This rising determination is becoming both stronger and more and more welcome. You are now finding more resources inside you than you ever thought possible. You find yourself richer in the ideas and the thoughts which inspire you.

(Name) You take a great pride and a great pleasure in the simple ease with which you *are* more enthusiastic and achieve more and more. Success is becoming easier and easier, enabling you to enjoy all that you do more and more, with each new successful experience you have.

(Name) Some people just call themselves average, but being average means that they are just the worst of the best, or the best of the worst. Such people never realise, that with even a modest improvement in their achievements it puts them higher up, and into the *top* half of performers and achievers. And that greater success *naturally* leads to further success.

Some people, who accept standards of less than their potential, miss much of life's pleasures and rewards. But, (name) you are *far* removed from such attitudes, attitudes that hold *others* back. On the other hand too (name) some people, even with little education or other advantages, go right to the top, and become eminently successful achievers.

(Name) you too have *every* natural facility to become a successful achiever. You have all the strength of purpose, determination and willpower you need. And in all that you do, every step forward makes the next step even easier to achieve.

You surprise yourself, even amaze and delight yourself, with the *simple* ease with which one achievement motivates the next. In all of this too, you have a lasting sense of pride and satisfaction, for you *are* a determined and successful achiever. Congratulations (name)!

TIMIDITY AND FEARS

In a moment (Name) I'm going to give you some suggestions that will

help you to be and feel stronger, more self-determined and purposeful. (Name) As I continue to talk your subconscious is beginning to realise, recognise and understand a simple fact. And this is, that you are actually more self-confident and outward looking than you thought you were in the past.

You see (Name) everybody is born to be self-confident and naturally self-assertive, and only through faulty self-programming can

this be eroded. Such programming can be reversed easily and quickly by discovering the truth. As you begin to see that you *do* have a greater inner strength, you find that you change. That you become more confident, and that you are becoming more and more the person you were originally born to be.

As I continue, I want you to imagine something; I want you to imagine yourself looking at a group of nervous, hesitant people. As you look at them you see how others can so easily dominate them take advantage of them, and intimidate them. Some of them appear even fearful in some way, as if frightened, perhaps over one thing in particular, or possibly fearing some general situation.

As you continue to imagine these people you realise they are the victims of their fears because they are the victims of themselves, of their own *imagined* weakness. Even though they may be physically strong such people never realise they are under-valuing themselves, or they create their own invented fears, making them become a reality.

(Name) now imagine a second group of people, some may be weak and feeble physically but see how they are certainly very confident, determined and forward looking. They know what they want and expect, they think and behave in a purposeful and positive way, their feelings, reactions and thoughts make the way they are a reality because they see the positive response and respect that they command simply by their positive attitudes.

Such people remain undaunted, unselfconscious and unintimidated; they enjoy the rewards of their positive thinking and determined reactions. For them the quality of life is higher and more satisfying. They never stop to consider why they are as they are; it is simply the result of allowing themselves to develop in such a positive, rewarding and self-enriching way.

(Name) just by making the conscious decision to join that second group you have become stronger, more confident and more determined and assertive. You are becoming more able to express yourself freely and you are more at ease with yourself in all situations. It is as if you have just become more forward and hold things in a more realistic way but what is really happening is that you have simply re-discovered your own natural inner strength so that coping and dealing with things in a confident and competent manner is just the natural way you are.

For you are confident, determined and assertive, expressing yourself well, reacting in a relaxed, self-assured sort of way that delights and even impresses you with how you always command the respect of both yourself and the others around you.

To be added to a recording that you intend to play frequently

(Name) Every time you hear this message it becomes more and more taken up by your subconscious, reinforcing all the amazing, and enjoyable effects that are even now taking shape and form within you. For you are now *taking charge* of your life, and confidently play the leading role in it, as this was always your right from the very beginning. (Name) You are now going from strength to strength, and in all of this, well done.

STRESS AND ANXIETY

(Name) You are relaxing more and more, and you are feeling more and more peaceful. As I speak, your mind and body are beginning to run in total harmony together, more and more. An inner feeling of peace and tranquility is flowing into every part of you. You are relaxing more and more with every word that you hear, and with every breath you exhale a wonderful feeling of quiet inner peace and tranquility, as if a warm inner glow of personal harmony is developing within you. You're just letting go, and relaxing.

(Name) As you experience these wonderful feelings, your mind is enjoying them too. As your mind enjoys them, it adopts them, by keeping and retaining them, so that being calm and relaxed are becoming natural habits, and all just the way you always are. With these good feelings of calmness and relaxation you find an amazing capacity to cope easily. You find yourself feeling happier, far more content, taking everything in your stride, easily, comfortably, competently and well.

(Name) You sleep better, sleeping soundly each and every night. You are becoming more cheerful, seeing and realising more of the pleasures and joys in life. You think more positively and clearly, and feel more and more relaxed on every occasion. (Name) You are at peace with yourself, relaxed, confident and calm. These feelings are more and more felt and enjoyed with every day that passes. Each day you simply become, and remain, calmer and calmer, more and more relaxed, with the peace and quietness that you now have inside you.

PREGNANCY AND CHILDBIRTH

(Name) I'm going to give you some helpful suggestions, suggestions that will help you to relax more, and as you relax more, help you to feel better too. (Name) For you do find that you are relaxing more and just feeling good. - That a warm inner feeling of peace and harmony is developing in your mind, bringing confidence and inner tranquility.

You are now finding everything easier than you may once have thought it would be, because, by the very nature of relaxing, your body performs more smoothly and efficiently. Leading you to feel more comfortable and at ease. Everything is going well, and you look forward to the arrival of that miniature human, eagerly needing the love and protection you give.

(Name) You find yourself feeling more confident, sleeping better, feeling fitter, and feeling happier and more fulfilled as a woman. You are now experiencing the good emotions and successes that you will look back upon as wonderful experiences, and experiences that you treasure forever. You are feeling good all over, healthy, fit, happier and more content. You take a great pride in your pregnancy, and how well it all goes, and gain great confidence, from all the modern expertise that is now there, to help and support you.

(Name) You are delighted with your progress, looking forward to the coming event, of having your child in your arms, to love, kiss, cherish and to have. A fulfilling experience you've so often dreamt of and wanted. Your mind knows all that it needs to, to help you and your baby do well, so that your mind relaxes your body, and makes the arrival of your baby a satisfying and fulfilling experience - and all with the natural timing that is perfection.

You amaze yourself at how at ease you always are, and how delightfully simple it all goes. You are increasingly confident, and taking all in your stride. You are proud of yourself, proud of that small child, and delighted that everything goes so well. (Name) Congratulations!

HYPNOTHERAPY AND SEXUALITY

This chapter is designed to help the reader understand sexuality and how the various aspects or inclinations can arise with the hope that such understanding will help the reader to deal with any issues that are troubling them.

Second only to self-preservation, sexuality is our most powerful driving force. In one form or another it intrudes into our lives and in a wide range of ways, bringing with it much of what we are as individuals. So enormous is it as a subject that it is only possible to look at it in the way it concerns those who wish to use the enormous power of hypnosis, for self-help and understanding. For our purpose, it is only necessary to grasp the basic concept that sex is an enormously powerful force. That it remains under the control of the subconscious and is governed or restrained to a socially acceptable level by the conscious. We need to understand that the sexual inclinations, responses and reactions that develop are the products of our upbringing and experiences. And that attempts to suppress our sexuality lead to anxiety and neurosis.

Although the powerful sexual drive that we have is equal in both male and female, it expresses itself and responds in different ways in each. While the male is more easily aroused and responds to sexual situations mainly through visual effects and seeking physical gratification, the female responds to sexuality more through emotion, romance and love. Both sexes however, have physical and mental gratification needs.

It is as if we are born with minds largely neutral or blank - other than for those inbuilt genetic factors which are going to run our bodies as if by some automatic process. Only very gradually as we evolve over our first few months and years, will our intellectual conscious mind come to have a greater effect on our developments and reactions.

Initially we start at the same applied intellectual level as any other animal. It is our developing intellectual response to our experiences that is to make us become, not only what we become, but separates us so widely from other animals. During these early years we are extremely vulnerable to misunderstanding things, and making mistakes - both mentally and physically.

As adults it is difficult to understand the naive perception an infant has of the world around him, as he develops into his early childhood. But those wishing to understand the mind, to the extent required to enable good hypnotherapy to proceed, need to meet this fundamental requirement, and particularly in the sexual aspect. Both the male and female child is usually brought up initially and primarily, by their mother. To each, the mother represents nourishment, love, security and entertainment. To these the male will add sexuality. Not in the adult sense, but deep down subconsciously, and in an infantile way.

As a result of his subconscious sexual awareness he will have reactions, such as experiencing erections that will be just as real to him as they are in the mature adult. However, with a limited intellectual contribution these reactions will be vulnerable to distortion, and as will be explained in the chapter on the complexes, this is going to have a potentially enormous effect.

Eventually the developing boy is going to become aware of the role of his father, who will be seen subconsciously as a rival for his mother's love and attention. His brother too, is likely to be seen in this role, with his subconscious becoming aware of the challenge for the mother's love and attention, and will often recall its great concern and the perceived potential peril in its dreams. Commonly, the boy will have a repeating dream of being chased, but never caught, with the mind concealing the real source of the threat by representing father (or brother) as a bear, lion, wizard or even as the unknown.

The boy may dream of being chased but never looking back so never knowing by what. He may dream a cupboard contains some evil monster, which could come out and into his room at anytime, but in the dream it may never actually do so. The boy may wake if he is confronted by his father or brother in real life.

The father or brother is never consciously aware of his possessive competition for her; his father's wife or brother's mother.

The female child will experience similar conflicts because although she loves and needs her mother, she too is eventually to become aware of that father figure, who is sometimes there, sometimes not, he is perceived as 'shadowy' figure, who has a great influence on her mother. The father becomes almost dangerously tempting, intriguing and exciting to her subconscious. She feels helplessly drawn to him and risks the security and love of her mother by turning to him.

In her dreams she may see herself in some dangerous situation or under some mysterious threat. Commonly, and as with the male, she may dream of herself being persuaded by a witch (her mother in disguise) and being chased for her disloyalty and for competing for the mother's partner. However, because her initial prime human contact is with her mother, who is of course of the same sex, she is to remain sexually neutral or sexually unawakened during her earliest stages when, as with the male infant, she is most vulnerable to misinterpreting experiences.

Despite this delay, eventually her subconscious needs for sexual expression and experiences will arise and occur. When it does, it may happen independently of the male figure. Sexual pleasure may be experienced, although the little girl doesn't consciously know that it is a sexual experience. Since such experiences are mostly devoid of a male's presence, occurring as if by accident the girl will have the tendency to continue to remain sexually neutral.

As a result she will develop with fewer, if any sexual deviated orientations. Consequently, later on she will need more stimulation to become sexually aroused. Because her basic subconscious needs for sexual experience continue to exist, in the absence of stimulation it will 'boil over' at times.

However, with the need of stimulation for sexual arousal, together with her inbuilt fear of the consequences of a premature pregnancy, the female will be able to defer her sexual activity more easily than the male. Once her sexuality is triggered she too will find sex as irresistible as males, but have a greater capacity to control it. She may even withdraw her sexual needs and return to those she experienced in early childhood.

To the female child, her father's voice identifies him as a male, and becomes part of her attraction to him. Subsequently a man's voice is to play a large part in her choice of partner. In fact some say that while the male falls in love with his eyes - and assumes that all else is secondary to what he sees - the female to a lesser extent falls in love with her ears.

Women, far more than men, will be heard to remark on a man having a good, lovely or horrible voice. This factor also plays a large part in the female generally being the predominant listener, and the male being the predominate talker in relationships.

Because the female child initially develops a neutral sexuality it helps her considerably later to smooth her path to adapting more readily to the male who comes into her life.

Partly from the leadership given to her in her sexual relationships, and partly from the experiences she has had as she has matured, the female will adopt her own sexual tendencies and reactions. It is as if her sexuality arrives with experiences acquired in maturity, rather than from early immaturity and naiveté.

Unlike the girl child, the boy has been brought up in an environment with frequent sexual encounters. His mother is female, and becomes increasingly apparently so to him. There are the essential physical contacts of dressing, washing, and bathing him. His mother, unintentionally, will constantly arouse him sexually. Time after time he will experience an erection for her, without him consciously realising it is directed to his mother. Although the mother may be amused or puzzled by his erections, most mothers have no idea that the erections are the product of sexual feelings being directed toward her, by her son's subconscious. She will be seen by him in her various states of undress and at times heighten her presence by dressing-up, wearing make-up and perfume.

All of this will be registered by the developing boy's mind, both consciously and subconsciously. If the boy has a repeated, or even a single sexual experience which is sufficiently sexually arousing, the male child may link that experience directly with his sexuality. This often results in him adopting a fetish, preference or an unusual sexual reaction. This may not only take hold of him at even a very young age, but persist as a powerful influence for life. Suppose the mother, either on one occasion or repeatedly, appears in say, shiny underwear, and the male child is or becomes subconsciously sexually aroused, he may then add what he sees in his mother's clothes to his mothers sexuality, and then add this to his own sexual arousal.

Subsequently a sexual fetish or preference for such clothes or materials could emerge, although he will normally remain unaware of its origins. This may then be extended to the developing male's need for sexual satisfaction, with him only being aroused by similar underwear, or give rise to transvestite tendencies. Where such tendencies are more acutely felt, such a person may cross-dress openly or secretively, in many cases unknown to his wife, or ultimately be driven on to desire a change of sex.

Although less common, similar reactions of cross-dressing occur in females, but where they do, are more likely to have other factors playing a part, Lesbianism, the simple extension of tomboyish tendencies or just for convenience, for examples. Although transvestites are mostly heterosexual, transvestism is often to be found in homosexuals. In either case narcissism is at work, transvestism being a self-satisfaction need, is self-indulgence by nature. Probably half of the male population has indulged in some form of transvestic experiences. Mutual 'cross-dressing' can also be of a bisexual nature, in which case it is as much of a partnership need rather than being self-satisfaction based only.

Females too, can experience excitement and sexual arousal from dressing up. However, this is because she sees her clothes as an addition to herself or as an extension of her sexual display, and her arousal comes from heightened sexual anticipation, and not so much from the clothes in themselves. The clothes are a means to an end to her rather than an end in themselves. Clothes to a woman are an essential reflection of her as she is, wishes to appear and feel. Dressing well can give much added self-confidence but especially to a woman, even if like underwear, it may never be seen by another. I know of at least one woman who always wears stockings and a suspender belt on important occasions like meetings and interviews, but at no other time.

Returning to our male child for a further example of sexual distortion, supposing he is sufficiently sexually aroused while being bathed by his mother, with her wearing a plastic apron. Under such conditions he may link the sensation he experiences by touching the apron to his sexual arousal. He may emerge with a sexual reaction or fetish to rubber or leather, having subsequently encountered these materials, and mistakenly taken them for the material that he associated with that earlier sexual experience. Of course, instead of it becoming rubber or leather it could have remained plastic itself.

As yet a further example of an origin of sexual deviation, take a situation of the more prudent mother. The boy sits in the bath and is sexually aroused; he puts his hand on his penis, the centre of his reactions. The mother now chastises him, possibly heightening his reactions. The mother then forcibly removes his hand, holding it firmly behind his back, the arousal continues and the boy now employs his other hand causing the mother to similarly hold the boy's second hand behind his back.

The boy wriggles, attempting to free himself to indulge his sexual arousal and touch his penis again, but now with a sense of excitement and challenge developing. Given such an experience both participants are likely to find similar situations arising on subsequent bathing occasions. If the original reaction had been strong enough, following such experiences, a bondage inclination might emerge later in life, where he may seek pleasure from being bound or inflicting it on others.

Similarly, masochistic tendencies will have their origins in early behavior and parental reactions of the time. Sexual deviations can also result from encounters with other family members, particularly between brothers and sisters, and when they do, may become depravations. For instance, the young brother becoming sexually aroused by the sight of his younger naked sister could link his sexual inclinations to young girls.

Should this occur, as his sexuality develops, he could find that young girls sexually stimulate him, and he may even be driven on to seek sexual intercourse with them. Equally, should he experience a stimulation of a similar kind in the presence of a male child, he might also develop a craving for sexual acts with young boys. In rare cases the female can be stimulated in this way, causing similar reactions to those of the male.

In homosexuality we have other factors at work, and these can include genetics, reincarnation or experiences during development. Where homosexuality is the product of subconscious mind programming or as a result of events in life, it will tend to be a narcissistic neurosis (love of oneself).

In principle, the narcissistic homosexual really wants to make love to himself, but cannot do so. In expressions and acts they are demonstrating what they really expect and need to find in their partner, but being directed to them. The intently self-inwardly looking nature of this neurosis often results in the need for a high number of partners, particularly so with males. For what is sought cannot be found - that is, himself as his partner.

This often leads to experimenting and searching. It is this unfulfilled need in two individuals who each turn their own sexuality inwardly and onto themselves that often lays at the heart of the many relationship difficulties experienced by such partners or couples.

Another origin of homosexuality, some say the most single origin, is where, from an early age, the male child desperately seeks the his fathers' attention, approval and love, perhaps in competition with this mother. When this need is not sufficiently responded to, as seen by the boy, his subconscious will continue to yearn for it. He 'loves' his father but feels he has not had that love returned and continues to want and need it.

As the child grows the original need remains in the subconscious and requires fulfillment. He must look for another male to fulfill that need. He becomes the homosexual needing a father-like or dominating partner. When one is found he is likely to prove loyal to that partner. Following analysis, this homosexual may gradually return to heterosexuality, especially where, as is most common, he was heterosexual prior to becoming homosexual.

Another sexual variation the experienced hypnotherapist will encounter is the transsexual.

Transsexuals are mostly poles apart from homosexuals. Although transsexuals are very often driven by transvestic tendencies, by definition they are rarely homosexual, having any tendency towards their own sex, or choice of clothes, only as the natural extension of their changing sexuality. That is, the transsexual changes sides as well as gender.

The lesbian can derive her sexuality from a source not too common in males. If during her early childhood the natural love between daughter and mother is not detracted from by a significant presence of a male figure, then the girl's developing sexuality is left with nowhere else to point itself, and consequently the natural loving bond can take on a sexual connotation from the need of sexual expression. The stage can be reached, where the time of becoming 'converted' to heterosexuality is passed. This sexual orientation may well remain within the subconscious even if suppressed by the conscious, to emerge later as a lesbian tendency.

Alternatively if the father is present, but at the time her sexuality should have developed toward him, she is to realise that he is in some way undesirable, then the transfer of her sexuality from her mother to father may not occur. The female under such circumstances, may become bisexual - a sort of 'half transition having occurred.

A further variation of possibilities is where the female infant subconsciously feels herself, not competing with mother for her father's love and attention, but rather with father for her mother's love and attention. In this case she may develop anti-male tendencies, should she feel that she has lost that competition.

In general, few fathers really understand how important they are to their daughters. That is not to say they do not love them or that they neglect them, but rather, in many cases, they have either never realised it or understood it. A father's love is needed to be seen and demonstrated to her. The daughter has an essential need to be told that she is loved by her father, needed, intelligent, clever, bright minded, talented, pretty, lovely and adorable.

The father must find the time and make the effort to show sufficient interest, participate, encourage and applaud his daughter. The 'you know I love you, so I don't need to say it' carries no weight or conviction. The love has to be expressed! For the little energy and effort required, the benefits will present a rich harvest of happiness for all. In this expression, sons too require their share. Not the least of all, a wife needs it too.

Whatever their sexuality or tendencies the person will prefer themselves as they are, although coming to terms with homosexuality can be a very difficult process, with the subject feeling highly confused, at least initially, or feel embarrassed, self-conscious and certainly unsure. Most will live with their secret closely guarded for years, even life. Some will enter heterosexual relationships hoping that it may in some way settle the issue, only to find in many cases, that secretive and socially risky homosexual encounters cannot be resisted.

In women, the need for security and the natural desires to bear children will be additional factors in seeking heterosexual relationships. In general the female will tend to hide her true feelings more successfully than men. Quite without knowing it or having any grounds for suspicion, some men and some women may live a contented and fulfilling life, never suspecting the basic homosexual orientation of their partner.

The experienced hypnotherapist will constantly come across a very wide range of fetishes, orientation tendencies and sexual experiences in clients, mostly in males, but in females too. The infant female will experience sexually arousing events, and, just as the male may do, identity her feeling with some tangible external factor. As a result she may develop a fetish or attraction for some masculine feature. The male's 'bottom', his ankles or his tie for example. These tendencies will be as compelling to her as the male's are to him.

In one case, for example, a female client said she had experienced a series of disastrous relationship with men, all of whom regularly wore silk ties. She was helplessly drawn to men wearing such ties. After speaking to me about it she asked her father if he had worn silk ties and he confirmed that he had always worn them. However, she was offended by my suggestion there could possibly be a connection and refused analysis.

In another case, a female client reported that she regularly watched snooker on television, to observe the players' bottoms (butts) as they leaned over the table to take their shots. She also reported that when alone she became sexually aroused by pinching their bottoms on the screen.

The above explains the processes most infants go through as a result of confusion and misunderstanding by the subconscious mind and the results that can often occur, however, as we know, the majority of children grow up and mature as perfectly normal sexually as their conscious and subconscious minds resolve the issues and misunderstandings quite naturally.

The following explains sexual deviations and fetishes and how they can develop as a result of the Electra and Oedipus complexes. These complexes and how to resolve them will be explained in detail later.

AUTOEROTIC ASPHYXIATION

This is a practice that kills around four males each week in Britain alone. The victim of the act is driven on to experience a situation of self-asphyxiation. In some cases hanging is the chosen method, but without the intention of dying. In others, self-strangulation or suffocation might be employed to achieve a similar objective, but again without the intention of dying. Often as part of the precautions some object, such as a tangerine, will be placed in the mouth to help keep an air channel open should the victim temporarily pass out.

Since I have never actually encountered a client with this condition, and have only met the family members of some men who suffered this condition, I can only speculate on the origins of the tendency. It is possible to imagine a situation where as a small boy, so terribly upset that he loses his breath, and while he continues to have difficulty in breathing, is intensively sexually aroused by his concerned and sympathetic mother. If this happens, he could have grown up having linked that difficult breathing experience to his sexuality.

Indeed, during early childhood, following an initial experience, he may have contrived to repeat the experience, and if he had succeeded this would have compounded his desire. Whilst this is all speculative theory, nevertheless evidence of a sexual connection is often found, when the activity does result in death - usually in the form of nakedness or female clothing.

SEXUAL MOLESTATION

As much as a daughter, not having had love from her mother, may lead her to find difficulties in truly loving her own daughter, a boy beaten by his father may find himself with a similar beating tendency towards his own son. In just the same way the child that is sexually molested or interfered with may have that tendency to interfere with his own children in turn. In some cases however, the sexual molesting can also have its origins in early experiences between children themselves.

Whatever the origins, the fundamental cause of the temptation, either carried out or not, is basically the same. The subject has had his subconscious programmed by events to act or think in a sexual way towards children. While the faulty programming may vary, in some way it will remain, and in some cases give great distress to the subject, while being either a potential or actual cause of enormous suffering to others. Added to this are all the prospects of the terrible consequences for the offender too, should the temptation be yielded to.

Where the temptation does overcome the resistance of the conscious mind of the perpetrator, it threatens to pass the tendency on like some terrible infectious disease. The perpetrator, or potential perpetrator, should always, I repeat always seek help, and preferably from a competent hypnotherapist, particularly a therapist using techniques at least similar to those set out in this book. In this respect, it should be borne in mind that not only is such therapy highly confidential, but is not entered, under current UK law, on personal records.

Sexual interference with children, particularly by males, is probably much more common than is realised, and causes much misery and resulting in ruined or badly distorted lives. Child sex abusers receive less sympathy for their behavior than from almost any other neurosis. Should they end up in prison, they frequently find themselves the butt of their fellow inmate's detestation, both verbally and physically and yet, of course, it is a neurosis.

The child abuser is as vulnerable to carrying out his activity or inclinations as any other neurotic sufferer is to his, and is helplessly trapped by it. As such he is deserving of sympathy. **Unless such a person realises help is available, but refuses to take it, preferring instead to remain as he is.**

In treating child abuse cases, it should also be borne in mind that intelligence, the left/right brain balance and the persons character all play a part in it.

SEX AND WATER

A curiosity, encountered by the therapist from time to time, is the various sexual connections that occur with water. People masturbate and copulate in baths and showers, enact fantasies with nocturnal swimming - often followed by copulation. A water bed generally produces more sniggering and innuendoes than any other type of bed.

Some people become sexually transformed in public toilets, more so men, where water and genital reactions come together. People dress in clothes termed 'wet-look' and some men will gain great satisfaction in looking at pictures of women who look as if they have just climbed out of a pool, and many women also find satisfaction in similar pictures of men.

Notice how frequently running and splashing water, sea, lake and river views are incorporated in advertising. Fishing, which combines the strong hunter challenge with the water environment is not only a major industry in its own right, it is also the biggest participatory sport in the country. Satin not only looks similar to the beautiful shimmering surface of a lake, surface, it also heightens the female physical form provocatively, and possibly because of this, it has become psychologically associated with sex.

Water's sexual stimulating effect probably goes back to those bathing sexual experiences that both males and females so frequently had in their early development. In fact water does have a very real sexual connection.

MALE/FEMALE REACTIONS TO DISADVANTAGE

Where the female encounters a man in some weakened state she will often have a natural tendency to mother him. Where the male comes upon the female in a weakened state, he will be tempted to take advantage of her vulnerability. Some cartoons depict this, and show the caveman, club over his shoulder, dragging his newly 'acquired' female along by her hair. This temptation can be experienced across the entire male spectrum.

Where the weakened or vulnerable female is encountered, and the male is unaware of the powerful subconscious processes involved, and succumbs to the temptation to take advantage of it, matters can quickly become out of hand. Given these circumstances the male will see the vulnerable female as an easy conquest. Every woman knows the risks of accepting an offer of a lift from a male stranger, for in so doing, she demonstrates her weakness through need.

A similar situation is even more likely to occur when the female is significantly weakened in her defenses by alcohol, and especially when her partner's inhibitions have been reduced by the same means. Rapes are constantly reported, that have resulted from seemingly innocent beginnings. The offer of the lift for example, may start with a genuine gesture, but those male forces can quickly take over. Subsequently, the male may say 'I didn't mean to', or 'I don't know what came over me'. Sometimes the outcome of the man's reactions to the woman's weakened state can be tragic and even fatal.

In the circumstances, the male's subconscious forces can quickly take over, and once the first sexually orientated advance is made it leads to another, and then another. In response to the female's refusal to respond 'positively' to the advances, the male can become angry, for in a way his subconscious cannot understand it. Ultimately, in order to conceal a situation that has lead to a given point, the aroused non-intellectual animalistic mind of the male may cause him to attempt abduction and/or even murder to cover his tracks, and all this quite out of character of the man's normal behaviour.

Fortunately for males, simply being aware of the principles involved is enough to check and override these natural impulses to act in this aggressive way.

The same subconscious forces, though far milder, can be experienced in the treatment of women by professional male therapists in all branches of medicine, including psychiatrists.

However, as previously put forward, by consciously being aware of the forces at work, no effort is required to over-rule them.

Interestingly though, the female will often have fantasies of having some male helplessly in her control, but luckily for men, the fantasy is mostly to remain at that. An alternative fantasy that some females have, is the one in which they are forced to surrender to a male in some way.

However, more often than not, the reality of such a situation occurring would quickly terminate any future such fantasy.

MASTERBATION

In masturbation we have mostly a normal self-fulfilled sexual relief, practiced by both male and female, and more commonly experienced during the earlier stages of oncoming sexual maturity. Masturbation is more common in males because of the greater ease with which male sexual arousal can occur. In fact, the most frequent form of sexual act occurs between those selling sexual services and those purchasing them are principally of a masturbatory nature. Hence some of those advertisements for massage services, with the emphasis on the attractive qualities of the masseuse. Those males taking up these services are mostly looking for an effortless non-involvement and speedy release of their sexual needs, in the excitement of the company of the female.

With the prostitute, the male will say and do things that he never would with his wife, because his inhibitions are quickly lost in the presence of someone not having to be lived with, or faced the following morning at breakfast. What he should know is that his wife might just as well have been the appreciative recipient of those same words or deeds, and which could have strengthened their marriage

Eroticism is often much enjoyed by the female, especially where the male lives up to the role of being a good husband in the marriage as a whole. What can be said for sexual enjoyment through eroticism with the prostitute or wife, can be said for any other sexual relationship too.

Masturbation normally causes little harm, but with some exceptions. Where it is a frequent and a solitary function, and only thoughts and visual aids serve as sources of inspiration, inevitably these can lose their attractiveness, leading to an increased search for greater stimulation. A course might then be set, in which considerable deprivation could result. Being discovered in the act of masturbation may well result in acute embarrassment, guilt or rage, and even result in the distortion or distraction from subsequent sexual relationships.

Similar feelings or reactions can also arise in those witnessing the act. Alternatively, the witness might be inspired to participate in some mutual sexually active response, and particularly where this occurs in a same sex situation, considerable mental harm may subsequently arise. Another possible negative effect is that the masturbator may adopt an acute sense of self-detestation, feeling different from others, or simply feel ashamed of giving into the urge. These feelings can occur in the woman, who has masturbated to the image of her father, or another close associate of her teens.

FRIGIDITY

Frigidity is a term given to a female condition, in which the sufferer is unable to derive pleasure from sexual intercourse. Frigidity either causes the inability to arouse a clitoral enlargement (the female equivalent to the male's erection) or produces a situation where clitoral enlargement is easily lost. Sexual ignorance of either or both partners may give rise to frigidity. Where the male suffers repeated premature ejaculation, or, where following insufficient foreplay, the male reaches his climax too quickly for the female to become sufficiently aroused to reach her orgasm, can also contribute to, or cause frigidity.

The frigid female often regards sexual intercourse with displeasure and where it is not brought on by a sexual partner other reasons need to be explored. It might be that conscious or subconscious reactions to sexual matters underlie it. Or perhaps faulty sexual education gave rise to the concept of sex being dirty, sinful or to be feared, and such feelings may then either contribute to or be the basis for frigidity. In some cases, sexual intercourse can be found to be painful - if so, a medical examination and treatment are called for.

Most commonly, psychological forces are at work. Sex may have been the subject of parental disapproval, or rejected on religious grounds. Badly conducted sexual experiences may also account for it. So too, having being caught in some sexual act or having been sexually abused may have contributed to frigidity. As might her having been condemned for her responses by a partner, who castigated her as incompetent, unsatisfying, undeveloped physically or being in some other way undesirable.

A further possibility is that frigidity could be the result of her having been the victim of rape. Another complication resulting in frigidity is that sexual activity can give rise to highly emotive negative reactions, which can easily lead to faulty subconscious self programming and lead to sexual inhibitions. Since frigidity is far more likely to be psychological in origin, it responds well to analysis, which can be expected to give rise to a considerably increased capacity for sexual pleasure.

IMPOTENCE

This can have much in common with the casual effects of frigidity, except for one vital difference, and this is that consciously, the male is far more likely to be eager for sexual activity and satisfaction. Because of this, and particularly where the condition persists, he is the victim of endless frustration, self-doubt and feelings of inadequacy.

Impotency is often erroneously perceived with a sense of shame by the male, who may react in many ways. Often the victim will throw himself headlong into some intense activity, as if to emphasise his other aspects of masculinity. Alternatively he may never marry or he may even shun female company.

As has been said before, sex is under the control of the subconscious not the conscious. Where the subconscious considers sex or sexuality as unacceptable, then it will override the desires of the conscious mind, rendering sexual intercourse abilities either infrequent or impossible. Variations of impotency include partially successful attempts and the inability to climax, despite prolonged and intensely physical efforts. Medical checks should be sought.

One method that can help is to place a restriction, but not one too tight, such as an elastic band around the base of the penis. This approach can often help where the erection is only partially obtainable, or where no erection is normally created. Used in conjunction with stimulation by the female, a successful result can ensue.

Sometimes impotency will arise only under certain conditions or circumstances, like the absence of a fetish ingredient, after drinking too much alcohol, during emotional conditions, initially with a new partner, during some act of unfaithfulness or rushed sexual approaches for examples. Ultimately, impotency too can be expected to be found as psychological in origin, and as such can as equally well respond to analysis as frigidity can.

ORGASM LACK

This is often the result of the male's failure to cause sufficient arousal in the female, or to complete sexual intercourse too quickly for her. When sexual intercourse is conducted too quickly by the male, the female will often have little recourse but to complete her orgasm either openly or secretively. By the time the male has completed his contribution, the female may well then be sufficiently aroused and have passed the point where she could sexually return to neutrality. The lack of an orgasm can, and normally does have a highly frustrating outcome for her. It may lead to women seeking alternative partners, or it might undermine an otherwise good marriage.

Repeated failures of an orgasm may result in the female having or becoming to have much in common with frigidity.

Education, understanding and a restraint of the tendency to rush by the male are all promising courses for improvement. However, psychological causes as outlined for male impotency can also be the cause of orgasm lack, especially where the male is performing his part thoughtfully and lovingly. In this case the analytical approach is the more likely to achieve lasting beneficial effects, and for both partners.

PREMATURE EJACULATION

In some sense this is the inverse of impotency, and it can occur with the initial stroke of penetration or even prior to it. To a certain extent this can be explained by an over arousal or excitement felt by the male, and especially so where it occurs in initial or early sexual encounters. However, should this tendency continue then psychological factors are indicated and need to be unraveled by analysis.

There is no 'normal' time span for the duration of sexual intercourse, since a wide range of factors can exist on any given occasion, but between twenty and thirty penetrating strokes would be more usual in mutually satisfying sexual intercourse.

One method of slowing or reducing the tendency of premature ejaculation is to apply a desensitising cream to the penis head. However, the condition often resolves itself. Where self-resolution cannot be awaited, and should the condition last, analytical therapy is again called for.

SEXUAL SADISM

In this, sexual gratification or sexual pleasure and excitement are sought by inflicting physical or mental pain on a member of the opposite sex. Sadism is frequently directed to a specific area of the body, or runs a predictable routine course. (Animals can also be the victim of sexual sadism by humans.) Such activity can even lead to the deformity of another and in extreme cases, to the loss of life. Brutal murders for example, and especially where mutilation forms part of the act, can often have sadistic sexual motives as the driving motivation.

In lesser tendencies, the sadist may display an aggressive attitude towards sex, while immediately prior to the sadistic activity he may have behaved in a charming enticing manner - not unlike some Jekyll and Hyde behaviour. The perpetrator may have the inclinations, but keep them well hidden and await his opportunity to catch the unwary, when it is too late for the victim to escape. He may wait until some commitment has been made and gone into, such as marriage. Or the male sadist may restrict his activities to prostitutes.

In mental sadism, humiliation, mocking, swearing, abusiveness or belittling may be the selected expression. As with most sexual deviations the sexual sadistic is unlikely to present himself to the hypnotherapist for change, since he sees his activity as a source of pleasure he cannot perceive as something he could give up, that is until a more dramatic act or some ultimatum occurs, effectively forcing his hand. More likely than the sexual sadist, it is his victim that turns to the therapist, seeking to alleviate the consequences of their experiences.

In sexual sadism, it is as if sex is a frustration released through aggression, with the victim being reduced in stature or physically punished for causing the arousal which in turn, is subconsciously felt by the perpetrator as reducing him to a state of need, and weakened by his sexual dependency.

Because of their normally lesser physical abilities, females will be more likely to express their sadistic tendencies in a mental way, such as by humiliating their partner, being the teaser, by flaunting, by openly flirting, or resorting to the pleasure of bringing her partner to a groveling status, perhaps by leading him on in some way, and at the last moment declining to proceed further. Following sexual intercourse, the sexually sadistic female may urinate over the male, or make him 'pay' for his act in another way.

Where sadism is directed at a member of the same sex, similar acts may be perpetrated or attempted as between members of the opposite sex. In marriage the non-sadistic partner may initially go along with such acts, even enjoying the novelty of such eroticism, but will almost inevitably tire of it or come to fear it.

Where sexual encounters become reduced in frequency because of the fear, pain and/or humiliation, the sadistic tendency will often be heightened, or escape the control of the aggressor in the sexual encounters which do occur. Sadistic tendencies have their origins in early life, possibly having started with severe punishment for sex play, or where subconscious sexual frustrations have been experienced.

In some cases, the sadist has himself been the victim of sadistic acts, and is merely passing his experiences on. The sexual sadistic may be carrying out some act of jealousy or revenge, having seen earlier in life another enjoying greater privilege, love, understanding, sympathy, or benefits.

In some cases they may have been humiliated, rejected or made to feel inferior earlier in life. Sadistic tendencies are found in many people, and may not have sexual foundations such as the apparently normal teacher, parent or leader who derives pleasure from punishing or humiliating.

At least mild sadistic and masochistic tendencies are to be found in all of us. Without these, there would be little to laugh at in knock about comedy, we would lack interest in much of the news, and not be drawn to scenes of disasters. The origins of such tendencies can be uncovered by analysis, and then be intellectually resolved.

MASOCHISM

Rather than being the perpetrator of pain, humiliation and sexual aggression in another, in masochism the preferred victim is himself. Masochism is normally less dangerous than sadism, since the pain is borne by the person who desires it, and he will call for it to cease when the pain exceeds the pleasure it produces - unlike the dangers of sadism, where the victim may be powerless to resist or bring an end to it.

A masochist may require stimulation by flagellation - often of his buttocks - or he may prefer being reduced to groveling or humiliation, seeing himself as the victim/beneficiary of the degrading acts that he is rendered to perform or suffer. He may wish to be the vulnerable sex-slave to his partner. The masochist may be stimulated by wearing or pretending himself to be forced to wear female clothing of some exaggerated type or style.

In the mental form of masochism, some may wish to be mocked, bullied or abused for their efforts. In both sadistic and masochistic types extensive fantasizing may take place, serving to increase their practiced tendencies. In this too, we can see an individual who may have experienced sexual stimulation from corporal punishment, or humiliation in early childhood. The prostitute specialising in satisfying the needs of the masochist, may advertise her services by calling herself 'Miss Whiplash', or use some other similar title.

Masochistic tendencies are more easily put up with, but inevitably tend to convey a sense of guilt, humiliation or distaste in the non-sadistic partner. Conversely the acts and participation sought from the partner may degrade the second person to sadistic tendencies. For some masochists being beaten, whipped or humiliated, can not only be an essential prelude to sexual intercourse, but can even serve as an alternative. In another but milder form, masochistic tendencies can be expressed as martyrdom or self sacrifice.

BONDAGE

Bondage is really an expression of a sadistic or masochistic inclination, except confinement is the principal reflection. The intention is to create a sense of captivation or imprisonment, and produce a state of helplessness, vulnerability or humiliation, although pain and suffering may form part of it. A danger is that the person, in bonding another may become carried away with his now helpless partner and be urged on to acts beyond those originally intended, with even fatal results. Those feeling the need to engage in it are, in almost every case, driven on by consciously and subconsciously felt sexual needs. Analysis is again called for.

NYMPHOMANIA

This is the female's inordinate sexual drive for frequent sexual encounters, and it is the reverse side of the frigidity coin in many respects. Here an earlier sexually based experience - such as an Electra complex based need, has in some way formed a more specific need for sexual satisfaction, and one which in reality, can never be achieved. The nymphomaniac is subconsciously inspired to re-experience or complete that earlier event that has never left her subconscious mind.

Subsequently she is driven on in some vague search to be satisfied in a way that is no longer possible, for she no longer can go back to the original event, and consciously does not even know what it is. Where the female restricts her nymphomania to a single partner, he will be much taxed in coping with her if he wishes to ensure her faithfulness. Men often have fantasies about meeting a nymphomaniac. However should they do so, their fantasy may well quickly prove less attractive in the reality.

VOYEURISM

Voyeurism is a condition in which a person becomes sexually stimulated by looking at the genitals of the opposite sex, or watching the sexual activity of others. The condition is the reverse of 'flashing' or exhibitionism. In many cases voyeurism is accompanied by masturbation, or a gradual and protracted ejaculation or orgasm, rather as in a slow secretion process. Voyeurism often becomes preferred to sexual intercourse itself. This 'peeping- Tom' reaction can give great offence to people - such as women alone and courting couples. Because voyeurism normally stems from early childhood sexually stimulating experiences, it can successfully respond to analysis.

There is a sexually stimulating voyeuristic tendency in many people. Sexually explicit magazines, videos, and newspapers specialising in sexual scandal are various forms of this. The person taking this tendency to extremes covertly, or even overtly where possible, can make it their main sexual interest. Such people may go to great lengths, and show much patience and determination in seeking to satisfy their craving.

Voyeurs have been known to fall to their deaths trying to maintain or obtain a good position of observation. Mostly the voyeur in some way sees sex as something almost naughty or shocking. As a result, watching sexual behaviour rather than participating in it excites the voyeur to such an extent, that a husband may even prefer to witness his wife having sexual intercourse with another male, rather than being the participant himself.

FLASHING AND EXHIBITIONISM

These are two versions of the same basic condition. In their childhood, just when they are becoming more aware of life, some children also suddenly become aware of their sexuality and felt a need or temptation to share the novelty. More likely than not, those who develop the trait probably started to yield to the temptations of self exposure from around five to seven years of age. They experienced a naughty sense of fun in the criticism, chastisement, surprise or shocked reactions it produced in others, particularly members of the opposite sex.

A deep sexual pleasure may then develop from subsequent acts of exposure later in life. While such self-exposure is highly illegal, and can give rise to serious anxiety and anger to those exposed to it, most exhibitionists and flashers would become alarmed at the prospect of being punished for their actions. They are mostly inadequate personalities, both sexually and socially. The more stable woman, although upset and angered by the flashing male can usually cope, perhaps by kidding herself that she is amused by it.

A method of dealing with a flasher that was related to me by a client, and one that she found highly successful, was to respond to the flasher by bursting out laughing, and saying "If I had one like that I wouldn't show it to anyone!"

FURTHER NOTES ON SEXUALITY

Clients frequently consult hypnotherapists with sexual problems, these can be of a physiological nature as well as psychological. The therapist will have a very wide range of such cases being reported to him by clients. Especially since our sexuality often has such a powerful driving force that we are mostly unaware of, and because it is such an intimate subject, it is essential that the therapist should be very broad minded as well as being tactful in dealing with the subject.

A significant consideration that must be explored with people who have been sexually abused or raped is that at some point in the act, the victim of that act, in most cases, and if only fleetingly, will have experienced some sense of pleasure. Naturally such clients will regard any such sensation as unacceptable - even initially denying it.

This is completely understandable. Just imagine, for instance, the victim reporting such a matter to the police, and then adding that they had enjoyed some part of it. Any experience of pleasure should be looked for by the therapist, because it could be that aspect is causing a great deal of the victims suffering, and they are mostly unlikely to report it to the therapist voluntarily.

In sexual abuse and rape cases I usually bring the issue up along the following lines, having first discussed the incident therapeutically. "You know there's an odd thing about being human, and that is that we are driven on to have sexual experiences, and as part of that we are rewarded for those experiences with a sense of pleasure. It seems to be in our genes somehow. And it makes little difference to this response mechanism if it is an act we want or one we object to.

In many cases the rape victim, for example, will be totally baffled by having had a fleeting experience of pleasure at the time, and may then go on to feel upset and guilty, not realising that their reaction was triggered automatically and outside of their control. Tell me, where you a victim of that too?"

A further consideration, mostly with males and especially with those being molested after puberty age, is that they may take the pleasure experienced in the act as an indication that they are homosexual - or bi-sexual. As a result male clients in their late teens or twenties will consult the hypnotherapist confused about their sexuality and hoping the therapist will resolve the issue for them. In such cases the explanation of the origin of the pleasure factor must be included as part of that therapy.

Most rape victims will be very reluctant to report or even accept that any pleasure was experienced. Firstly one can hardly expect much by the way of understanding and sympathy from the person being 'complained' to as a victim, when the victim goes on to say that they enjoyed the experience in some way.

Secondly, and more importantly it is often felt as a great guilty secret that they, if they did, did enjoy part of the experience. In fact, where it exists, this sense of guilt may well be a major aspect of the client's concern. Subsequently it is often the therapist who has to explore this area, even bringing the matter up.

It is truly hoped that any rape victim reading this will now understand that any feelings of pleasure, even fleeting, is a natural reaction by the subconscious and not under the control of the victim, therefore the victim should understand that it is absolutely not his or her fault and there need be no feelings of guilt whatsoever.

Fortunately, with tact, this is not difficult, and in the way of proceeding to follow, no suggestion is made to the client that they did enjoy the experience, because such a suggestion could create a sense of guilt where none previously existed, say in the client that did not recall any sense of pleasure. Here's a good method of dealing with the issue, and normally following the client having completed the report of their experience.

Therapist. You know there's an amazing thing about sexual experiences, deep down in our subconscious mind we are driven on to perpetuate the human species through reproduction - all creatures are like that. The mind will normally reward our sexual activity with a sense of pleasure to encourage us. After all, if our sexuality was not rewarded in this way why would we bother?

Then the human race would decline and eventually disappear. Strangely, this primitive part of our mind knows or cares little about right and wrong, what should and should not be and tends to reward any sexual experiences with pleasures.

Without us realising what's going on this can happen even in cases where we feel greatly offended by some sexual encounter, and leave us perplexed that what's disliked still gave us a fleeting sense of satisfaction or even pleasure. When this does happen the victim may blame themselves in some way, or even feel immensely guilty, where in reality they were only tricked by their mind.

Following such a statement it is best left for the client to take this aspect of the matter up should he wish.

OVERCOMING RAPE OR ABUSE TRAUMA

A simple yet effective method is to use 'blow aways' to blow away the perpetrator and the actual event.

Another way is to imagine the perpetrator is in front of you and then say and do the things you couldn't do at the time, most likely you were young at the time, frightened and confused with no idea how to deal with the situation but now you are an adult and you do know what to say and do – do it now as you imagine that person in front of you, vent your anger, disgust and whatever else you feel, know that person was the victim of his or her own faulty programming, it is not an excuse, you cannot excuse the person but you can attempt to forgive. It will help then to blow him or her away.

Having a friend or a professional take you through the analysis, particularly the complexes is an excellent idea.

THE COMPLEXES

This chapter on the Oedipus and Electra Complexes you will give you a deeper understanding of how these sexual orientations and conditions can occur and very effective ways of helping people overcome them.

I need to explain that a symptom can arise, not from some consciously experienced event that is subsequently repressed and thereby hidden, but from a subconsciously produced experience, one that has its origins in the subconscious mind itself, and when this has happened it calls for a special approach, resolving the matter not through a conscious mind release but rather by dealing with it where it is.

The following procedure is most effective if the reader has a friend to play the part of the therapist by inducing hypnosis and reading out the following text. Alternatively, it may be worth considering visiting a professional hypnotherapist who has been trained in this procedure.

To do this I explain to the client that I must take the matter up in a way that the subconscious can easily understand, and to make sure of success I must put the issue forward in two separate ways.

I continue by saying, "What I am going to deal with soon, I go through with every client. In doing so with you I have no way of knowing if it is relevant or not" I point out that I shall not ask them to consciously accept it as relevant, but I do ask them to agree to keep an open mind. (Although the complexes have been covered previously, in what is to follow is the suggested method of conveying an explanation to the client, and as such is different.) To simplify the procedure I adopt, the method is given divided into parts.

Note: Parts one, two, three and four that follow must be interpreted by the therapist in accordance with the therapist's personality and in a way acceptable to the client. For no absolute script can be given that would always suit everybody. It is more essential that the therapist understands the principle involved than attempt to read out or memorise some script. In this way the issues can be adapted to the needs they are intended to serve.

From time-to-time during the presentation, it is also advisable to check with the client as to how they are reacting, perhaps by asking the client if they are following what's being said, or asking them to come in with any point they wish to raise, this will help keep the therapist in touch with the client's reactions.

In my years in practice, whilst the complexes have on occasion been rejected, they seldom are, and I have never had to terminate my presentation of them. In response to what little negative reaction does come from the client you have those statements you made before you began. You are presenting them with an opportunity of releasing a subconscious anxiety that could possibly have the most serious physiological as well as psychological consequences eventually, in addition to any symptom currently being suffered.

PART ONE, PREPARATION

I ask them if they were aware that a newly born male can experience an erection when less than an hour old. This, I continue, proves three things.

One, that sex is present from the very beginning, and since the sexual intensity is equal in both males and females the same can happen to the female infant, but would be less visible of course.

Two, that sex is under the l control of the subconscious, since while the intelligent conscious mind exists, it knows nothing at such an early stage.

Three, the reaction of the erection shows that the subconscious lacks intelligence, for if it had any, it would realise the reaction is fruitless. The reaction itself stems from the desire to copulate, and is a response to the preservation of the species reflex action, arising from the fear induced by the birth itself.

PART TWO, EXPLANATION TO MALE CLIENT

Now let's look at what's going to happen to the male infant. Over the first months and years, his mother is going to love him, wash him, bathe him, dress him, tickle him, take him out, talk to him, play with him, and feed him. Of course, his mother is female and he is male. What is he going to make of all this attention, her looks, smell, kindnesses, soft touch and understanding?

Why, that a special and highly attractive relationship exists between them, and of course all this with sexual overtones too, and with the intelligent conscious mind making little contribution. His subconscious is going to start arriving at its own conclusions and ideas. Namely, that his mother is his partner but bigger, more authoritative and cleverer than him, and that the gap must be closed. He must grow up and be seen as successful and more equal. He is subconsciously sexually in love with her, having an affair if you like.

Sooner or later however, he is going to become aware of rivals, in the form of sisters or brothers perhaps. However, there is one major rival he becomes aware of, his father.

Gradually he becomes more and more aware of the father, subconsciously resenting him and the advantages he has over him.

He may become subconsciously fearful of being found out by his father, and his subconscious might well reflect this in his dreams, where he pictures himself pursued or threatened. Indeed, his perception of being threatened may be more real than it is imagined, for his father may well, even if much later, subconsciously pick up the signals being transmitted by the son to his mother, particularly if, as they often are, similar signals are transmitted back from mother to son.

It must be emphasised, not only are both mother and son intellectually ignorant of what is going on, being left only with subconscious inclinations and feeling towards each other, but that each would strenuously deny any such allegation, especially in maturity.

However sooner or later, perhaps when he is packed off to school as if no longer needed at home, the son will perceive his battle as lost, although the subconscious programme is never cancelled, but just left as it is, with any of the thousands of possible permutations that may have resulted.

Those early emotions and experiences remaining locked into his mind will have changed him, and effect him for the rest of his life in many ways. This programming may remain undetected, even forever, or suddenly spring into effect in some way, with some experience or event yet to come.'

Following my explanation, I tell my client that what I have just described is called the Oedipus complex, and then, much as if some afterthought or in some casual sense of interest, ask "Do you think it may, in some way, have played a part in your life too?".

Where the response is one of doubt, I leave it at that because his subconscious will know the truth, and in bringing the mature intellectual reasoning and rational explanation to bear, the task of removing the effects of the complex are achieved in any case. Where the client is gifted with greater insight, and especially where the complex can more readily be seen as the cause of some important negative aspect of his life, I often discuss the subject in a way more relevant to his case and his experiences, before going on to the next part of the session.

PART THREE, EXPLANATION TO THE FEMALE CLIENT

'The female, following her birth, will be looked after by her mother, who will of course do everything for her. Showing her love, attention and kindness, she will dress, bathe, wash, kiss, tickle, talk to and sing to her. She will put her to bed, be with her when she awakes, and come when she cries out.

During all this her sexuality will come into action from time to time, and who is there to point it at, and be the object of it but her mother? But somehow it doesn't quite fit, there's something missing, the sexual aspect is not completely fulfilling, it's as if she needed something else.

The intelligent mind is of little help, the subconscious must make the most of the situation, while lacking the intelligence necessary to get things into perspective and draw accurate conclusions. The programme of attachment is laid down; she must close the gap between her and her mature, intelligent, authoritative mother, to secure the relationship in the satisfying way that it is currently felt and enjoyed.

As the weeks and months pass, she is to become aware of another figure in her life. That figure is a man (brother, uncle, grandfather or other) but most likely her father. He is different to her mother, slightly dangerous in a sense, but also mysterious, exciting and intriguing. All these reactions are going to incline her sexuality towards him, leaving her with a subconscious dilemma of choice between father and mother. A fascinating attraction to her father develops, that conflicts with the security she needs from her mother. She needs both, but feels that she must choose between them. Her subconscious is going to express her plight in its dreams. What if she were to be found out as it were, and then goes on to project this fear of discovery, by seeing herself pursued.

She may be pursued in her dreams by a witch or monster, yet never caught because she never is found out in the way she fears, but in another way, because she cannot help herself transmitting her signals of infatuation, and especially where these are returned, they will be intercepted by the mother. Without realising it consciously, the mother may now develop an attitude of jealousy or enmity towards her daughter later in life.

As an alternative response, or perhaps in addition, the daughter having lost the competition with mother for father's attention, she may be inspired by jealousy herself However, subconsciously the infant female may instead perceive the switch of her love from mother to father, as an act of disloyalty. As a result, a further conflict may arise, because the infant girl now wants to do everything she can to retain and secure her original relationship with her mother.

In all of these mental conflicts and desires, little intelligence is brought to bear, and subsequently her non-intelligent subconscious has to develop its own plans. She may decide on a never-ending expression of loyalty to her mother, and feel guilty for selecting her father as her choice for the time she did. Earlier she had programmed herself to go on trying to make the relationship with her father complete in every way.

If later, her father proves himself to have been unworthy of her intentions, she may grow to hate him, and desperately seeking a replacement that will give her the satisfaction she once sought. These early conflicts may continue to affect her in her future relationships and in many other ways too. In addition to all the possible permutations of reactions is to be added the greatest complication of all - that in the way it was originally intended to develop, her relationship with her father comes to nothing. She is ultimately going to have to exchange him for another male.

PART FOUR, PRESENTATION AND CONCLUSION

In presenting this adjust the male/female terms accordingly.

Continue thus: " To explain all this in a different way let's imagine you have a friend, one that you've known for years and that you meet from time to time. One day your friend greets you in an enthusiastic and excited manner. Your friend can't wait to tell you that they had met someone a few weeks ago that is 'out of this world', and begin to describe him/her." "Saying how they met, what they've done, what they are planning, and how truly wonderful he/she is, and how excited he/she feels. It's as if, for your friend, the world has suddenly opened up to them. Your friend is walking on air and is already deeply in love. From time to time you continue to meet your friend, always to hear the same enthusiastic subject eagerly talked of you've never known your friend to be so happy and radiant".

"One day, almost beside himself/herself with joy, your friend approaches you and can't wait to tell you his/her great news, they are to get married. In your friend's enthusiasm, you are repeatedly pressed to confirm that you will attend the wedding, to which you repeatedly agree. No fixed date has actually been concluded but this will be agreed that evening, and you are assured that your invitation will be in the post, to arrive the next morning."

Your friend then leaves to pass the good news to another friend. You've never known anyone so smitten by love, and you feel very happy for him/her. You are wondering just what this 'magical' prince/princess must actually be like. You can't wait to meet him/her.

Now, you have your wedding present to choose, new clothes to buy, you wonder what date will have been chosen, because you have a full diary yourself. Now you are caught up in this thing. Next morning you eagerly scan your post, but there is no invitation card amongst it. The next day's post arrives the following morning, but still no card. Day begins to follow day until a week has gone by. Still no card and you have not seen your friend either. Curious! The following week begins, and it too proceeds through its course, bringing no card or any meeting with your friend. Curiouser and curiouser! Now a third week begins to run its course, still no card, still no contact with your friend".

On the Thursday you meet a second friend, one that you also see from time to time. You explain your concern at not having seen or heard from your first friend. Your second friend responds that they are in the same position and are curious too. Your second friend tells you that the first friend usually goes to a bar or club on the other side of town for a sandwich lunch on most days, and suggests that it might be a good idea for one of you to pop in to see if your mutual friend is there, and to find out what's happening" .

You decide that you will go. Accordingly, the next day you arrive at the club. It is a bright sunny day, so that when you first enter your eyes take a few moments to adjust. It's quite a busy place and your initial inspection fails to detect your friend. As you begin to wonder if you should ask someone if they have any news, or knows anything, a door to a back room swings open as a customer passes through.

You catch a glimpse of what might be your friend, sitting in the corner of the next room all alone and looking greatly unhappy. His/her clothes look as if they have been slept in, his/her hair is a mess and his/her shoes muddy. As you approach you wonder what to say. Fortunately you are spared your concern for your friend is anxious to meet you and to pour out his/her grief. Your friend is now in a highly emotional state and tells you that it is all over, the romance is shattered and he/she is near suicidal.

You press for details. Why, what's happened? Your friend does his/her best to explain. It seems your friend's partner had never intended things should have gone as far as they did. It had been intended by the other partner to be a temporary, more casual thing but that as it unfolded, the other partner just couldn't bring himself/herself to say so".

The time was never right; there was never an opportunity to spare your enthusiastic friend's feelings. Somehow, it couldn't be done and the situation just snowballed and got entirely out of hand. Finally, your friend continues by saying that when the date for the wedding had to be chosen, the issue was forced to a critical point. It transpired that the partner was already married and that the spouse, who had been away, is due to return any day now."

Your friend says they know the spouse and that person is a really terrible type. Your friend has told everyone of the relationship so the spouse is bound to find out and will come looking for them. So, says your friend, I have lost the greatest love I have ever known and gained a terrible enemy too. I don't know what to do or how to cope, my life is in ruins. I have made a fool of myself. Your friend then continued in the same vein.

(Client's name) "If such a thing really happened it would indeed be a catastrophe for the victim involved wouldn't it? *(Agreement)* But let's swap the victim for you. So that it's you in the chair, and begin to run time back, so that instead of you being your age now, you become twenty, fifteen, ten, nine, eight, seven, six, five or four and imagine that the principles of what happened in the story, have just happened to you!"

"Can you see what an unprecedented disaster it would be, what confusing decisions and conclusions your subconscious could arrive at? The hopelessness, anger and guilt feelings you might have? How you might - with the subconscious having a perfect memory of it for life - become depressed, angry, begin to lack confidence or subconsciously go on to feel the pain and frustration forever? And see how that could lead to disastrous consequences for some bodily part, if quite unrealised by you that part began failing under the continuing stress. Do you think that this complex might, even just might have entered your life in some way, or degree?"

In response to your question the client may react in many ways, some will say "yes!" Some, "possibly." and a very few say "no!" - their response doesn't matter because it will come from the clients intelligent conscious mind, and in hypnosis your client's subconscious has listened and it knows the truth, and that truth is that "yes!" it did happen. But with your explanation of it, it is able to adjust and see things as they were then, and how they are now for the first time.

The effect of either the Oedipus or Electra complex on your client could have existed to any of a wide degree of depths, but it would mostly have been there, and your explanation will either have resolved it or triggered the resolution through a new understanding. Your explanation has been given and is to be found especially worthwhile in some seven cases out of ten. If your client was not significantly a victim himself, you have still given him information that could be of great value in helping him to understand those around him better.

If you are right, as mostly you will be, then you will have changed his life for the better and forever, although you will never know which client's they are, from time to time you will be saving their life too. I am satisfied that, above all else, the two complexes are prime causal factors that produce some unexpected heart attacks and many other serious conditions as well.

CONDUCTING THE ANALYSIS

The following analysis sessions are designed for those wishing to help others, they are not practical for self-help except part of session five and six.

If you wish to undergo analysis it is a good idea to have a trusted friend share this book so he/she can act as a therapist, you can also do the same for the friend.

Before beginning the analysis sessions let me remind you of some important details if you intend to use these techniques to help others.

Fist, remember it is important to use the clients' name frequently, better still, ask the client what name their friends call them, for instance, client's name may be James but his friends call him Jim – Jim is the name you should use.

Secondly, allow the client to feel he has control over the session, especially during the induction. Rather than dictate do this or do that let the client do things at his own pace, so instead of saying "close your eyes now" it is better to say "when you feel ready and comfortable allow your eyes to gently close" and wait for the client to close his eyes. Instead of saying "relax now" ask the client to give himself permission to completely relax. Also it is good practice rather than instructing the client to go deeper, relax more or suggest his eyes are feeling heavy etc. simply say "notice how you are feeling more relaxed" or "notice how your eyes are feeling heavy and you prefer to keep them closed" – words to this effect. This approach allows the client to feel in control and by using the words 'notice how' it lets the client choose his own way of following your instructions.

Thirdly, belief and expectancy has a huge bearing on your success therefore it is worthwhile increasing the clients' belief in you and the therapy and boosting his expectancy of success. Even with your first client you must exude an image of complete confidence and professionalism, giving the impression that you *know* this will work and that you are very experienced in your work. When things go wrong never apologise or show any panic, remain calm and behave as if this was expected to happen then continue in some way that will put the matter right and then proceed.

One further consideration: I use a converted bedroom in my home as a consulting room (cuts rental costs). However, with clients of the opposite sex I always check they are comfortable being on their own with me and offer the use of my lounge as an alternative – if the client is not comfortable with you therapy will not be very effective. As I stated earlier in the course, the subconscious can pick up 'vibes' and, although it has never happened to me yet, there is the slight possibility that a client may take an instant dislike to the therapist, if this happens, accept it and refer the client to another trusted therapist.

This analytical approach is designed to cover eight sessions, however, as the first four sessions are 'free association' they can be reduced to two or even one session depending on how the client responds. If the free association is reduced to just one session then the total number of sessions for complete analysis would only be five.

What has been set down so far has now brought us to the exciting and satisfying situation where your knowledge can soon be put to practical use. For now we begin the journey from theory to practice, and with all the amazing consequences of success that can be expected as a result. However, some points should be considered prior to that final transition. Conscientiously conducted hypnotherapy along the lines to be set out can do much good.

Treatment however, once started, must be continued with until the symptoms have been resolved, or terminated only following an extended attempt where little or no progress has been achieved, and continuation offers little apparent prospects. Inevitably, some percentage failure rate will occur. However, since the success rate from the therapy techniques given is high, you should be expecting at least an 85% success rate, even from the outset.

Where success eludes you following conscientious therapy, it must be the client and not yourself who has caused that outcome. If the same dedication is applied to all you work with, and that dedication works with some nine out of ten, then logic must have it that, in the case of the tenth client he, rather than you have brought that result about in some way.

In my experience, among such people are those who lack commitment. For instance, everything else rather than their appointment has priorities, with them rearranging appointments readily, perhaps seeing their attendance more as an inconvenience. So too are problems more likely where little or no financial commitment is made by the client, though this is less relevant among family and friends.

However, following the analysis methods set out, you will be seen to have made a genuine effort, so the client can do little to criticise the therapy. In all of my years as a professional hypnotherapist, I have never been confronted by a client asking for the return of his fees, or claiming that I have let them down.

Sometimes the client's subconscious will deliberately seek to disrupt or terminate treatment. Watch out for the client who often claims to be too ill to attend, or the client who interrupts sessions to enquire if the therapy is getting anywhere, or starts to throw doubts, not onto the therapist, but the general nature of the treatment, or repeatedly expresses the view that the therapy will not work for him.

In very rare cases, where the need of the subconscious to protect the client from resolving his problem by confronting it is strong enough, it will invent a reason. With its lack of intelligence, such a termination of treatment in the presence of the therapist can be bizarre in the extreme. Their invented reason makes sense to them, but is absurd to the therapist. The reasons can be as daft as the client claiming to not like the colour of your carpet or the shirts you wear.

Discussing these excuses with the client he will easily see how ridiculous the excuses are and will most likely understand your explanation of the subconscious`s unwillingness to help you recall the causal event. The client will then most likely continue with the therapy.

In practice it is not always necessary to recall the causal event in order to resolve the problem, it is quite possible to explain to the subconscious that the causal event is no longer important because the client`s circumstances have changed and in any case the past is over and done with and no longer important therefore you can ask the subconscious to release the anxiety perhaps through the medium of dreams or to just let it go and make the required changes without the client having to know what caused it.

Ways of doing this will be discussed in the following pages.

`Sod's law` or `Murphy`s law` states that early on in your work as a hypnotherapist, you will meet just such a client, or one that does not behave or respond in a way that you might expect and the experience might put you off. That would be a shame and a great loss. The benefits you will bring to humanity will have to be experienced to be believed and as I say, not least by yourself. The client has arrived and as most do, urgently needs reassuring. The client will almost always be apprehensive of you, himself, hypnosis and the methods you will be using. He will only have hearsay and the stage hypnotist to go on. He is only with you because he is desperate. He has probably tried everything else and it all failed! You are his last resort, while actually you should have been his first. The client does not expect to be cured, but he has to try.

In the more extreme cases he will take the view that he doesn't know what he has let himself in for, but desperation has forced his hand. He is with you, and initially, probably at least mildly terrified, even regretting he came. He has worked out what you will do to him and what will happen, and he doesn't much care for the prospect. He would almost as soon leave as stay. To him by arriving he has 'done it', God help him, for he has only himself to blame. Hopefully he has read your leaflet or come by recommendation for if he has he will feel easier.

For my part I dress informally and display a cheerful confidence while being attentive, courteous, kind and sympathetic. My priority is to put him at ease as quickly as possible. I reassure clients by saying such things as: "There is nothing to the sessions, all we do is talk. The sessions are easy and enjoyable".

If the person is in a highly emotional state, I interrupt my normal routine of first seeking details of them. If it is hypnosis itself that is causing the fear or apprehension I will tell the client that at this stage we do not need hypnosis and proceed as described in an earlier section. I will then carry out my normal introduction process while they are more relaxed in hypnosis. Additionally, I am perfectly happy should they seek the comfort, as many do, for them to have someone with them.

I shall want to know the client's marital or boy/girl-friend status. Do they have any children? What is or was the construction of the family they grew up in? Do they have, or have they had, sleep problems such as repeating dreams, nightmares, sleepwalking or talking in their sleep? What do they do for a living?

I ask for the details of any medication they may be taking which at an appropriate time I shall look up in a medical manual. For not only can their medication gives me some insight of their doctors' understanding and approach, but it can also help me to separate from his symptoms any adverse effects that the client might be experiencing from his prescription.

Although I will probably know before his arrival the nature of his problem, or it will be mentioned early in our initial meeting, I usually leave going into the details of it until I have the other information I need. There are several reasons for this. Going into details of their condition can often bring about emotional reactions, instantly hampering me in my attempt to gain a background, before plunging headlong into what might then have to be the start of the therapy, and thus leaving me to treat a client I know little or nothing about.

In such a situation confusing information can pour out in a torrent, leaving the therapist confronted with a tangle of detail. As an example, the client with relationship problems may present a list of disjointed and disastrous experiences with previous partners, leaping from one to the other - of course, while expecting the therapist to keep track.

Any misunderstandings or errant conclusions the therapist makes as a result of attempting to keep track of him may be seen by him as the therapist not understanding or following him. Then too, he will have questions he needs to ask, and you will also need to explain the procedures ahead, and you may need to reassure him regarding hypnosis.

You don't really want to be forced to induce hypnosis in the client before you have set the ball rolling if you can help it. Sometimes it is necessary, but I always feel that when hypnosis has to be induced as a priority, both parties are pitched in at the deep end. Fortunately, and despite what has been said, the client may not only want to, but also be able to discuss his problems rationally. Indeed this is mostly the case. However, I try to stick to my formula for the first session as far as I can, since the logical sequence reduces the risk of important information being overlooked.

My preferred routine in the first session, particularly with the more rational client, is to greet the client and put him at his ease, and then to ask for a brief indication of what he is attending for. Following this I seek out his background, and then return to his symptoms for further details. Of course, during this process I answer the client's questions as they are presented. Next I explain what it is that I expect of him.

When it does come to dealing with his symptoms with the more rational client, I go into some detail, such as asking when it started. Did anything significant happen in the two years preceding its onset? (You will recall that a repression can remain hidden until some other emotional situation is experienced, and that this secondary effect can bring into action the original repression. This having occurred, the emergence of the symptom can take from a day to up to two years to appear.) I probe this period in depth. Sometimes the client will be insistent that this secondary experience is the cause of his problem and the be-all-and-end-all of it too.

Where this belief is firmly held by the client, watch out for him expecting treatment to be specifically directed at it - a prerequisite of the 'are we getting anywhere' questions. I explain that a secondary situation often brings to light an earlier repressed experience, and it is this earlier experience that requires identifying and resolving.

Following this explanation, I hope to gain his willing co-operation in releasing that repression. This explanation is often necessary because the client will frequently say that such and such occurred prior to the emergence of his symptom, but then claim either that he has dealt with it, or that it is irrelevant because it was a happy experience: like being promoted, marrying etc.

On some occasions, a client will claim that what he needs is to be 'zonked out' and told to 'pull himself together'. The client will expect the therapist to go into details of his symptom because to him, as mentioned before, it has become the dominant thing in his life. However, as was also stressed earlier, any protracted discussion of his symptoms will hardly be of much benefit prior to hypnosis and therapy.

The client needs to understand that the resolution of his problem is to be found in its cause, not in the symptom itself, which is only the result. The client needs to understand that to do this he must commence the process by using 'free association', which I explain to him. It is also important to ask the client what he has done about his problem, for he may have been to a hypnotherapist before, and subsequently hold erroneous views in what he expects of you.

The client may have made several attempts to resolve his plight such as visiting a psychiatrist or undergone surgery. All of this information is always written down, and gives a considerable insight of your client before you proceed. Of course he expects you to show an interest in him and ask questions, so feel no reluctance in asking.

These techniques can be most useful, as well as reassuring and pleasantly surprising to the client, increasing his confidence in the therapist. Following all this I sit the client down and get him to relax into hypnosis, using whatever method seems the most appropriate for that client and the circumstances.

For what remains of the first session, following the induction of hypnosis, I will prompt the client to talk to me about himself and his life's experiences, often beginning by asking him about his earliest memories. In the process of free association, the client must be encouraged to say not only what he wants to say, as if as a relief like that from a confession, but everything else that comes into his mind. Even if it is disagreeable to him, seems unimportant, illogical, and irrelevant or is a repetition of what has been said before. Even if it seems ordinary, uneventful or something he clearly knows about anyway. In fact the benefit of free association is so enormous that, by using this method only, amazing results can be achieved.

Fortunately, many clients will take to the idea with enthusiasm and happily talk away. This is of course excellent, both for the client and therapist, for when the client is enthusiastically talkative he is off to a terrific start. At least as often however the client is reluctant to talk much, and where this happens I point out how essential it is that he should participate through talking, by explaining to him it doesn't matter what is talked about, because in talking he will give me information that he may not even realise will help me. Not only that, but talking about anything in hypnosis will exercise his mind in a way nothing else can equal, preparing his mind for the different work that comes later.

I also point out that in doing so his subconscious will learn that it can trust me. This is because, unlike normal experiences, I shall not offer advice, criticise, judge him, think him silly, tell him he's wrong, inadequate or suggest that he pulls himself together. Instead I shall listen with interest and because of that, trust will develop to the point where I can ask his mind to bring about change. Lastly I explain that in the course of free association, the root cause of his problem will begin to move nearer to his conscious threshold, making it much easier to release.

I sometimes illustrate this last benefit, by comparing it to the situation of a table tennis ball, hidden in a tub of corn. "You don't know where the ball is, but as you move the corn, the ball being so much lighter will bit by bit move towards the surface". (It is this factor that makes a premature termination of treatment unwise, because the symptom or the anxiety may become more pronounced).

Even with the explanations, the client may be reluctant to talk. If he is, I shall prompt him by asking questions about his earliest memories. How did his school life go? What about his early family life, his Christmas and holiday experiences and the like. Naturally, his chosen subject will often be his symptoms, and in which case I will let him carry on, since unlike the earlier situation, that is when initially talking to him to gain a background of him, he is now in hypnosis, and anything may be talked of. Subsequently, in talking about his symptoms, and without his realising it, he is already beginning to release them. This is because, unlike with just talking over his problems with a friend, his subconscious is now listening in and realising the consequences of his problems – problems caused by the subconscious itself when activating the repression.

Remember, this is for the first session and that other rules apply in subsequent sessions, in which, should he fail to 'burn himself out' of talking about his symptoms, he will need to be encouraged to talk of subjects other than his symptoms. In any case, symptom discussion should be restricted to the first two sessions. However there is a difference between his discussing the symptom itself, and his talking of his personal history in which the symptoms have played a role in his experiences.

Encourage the client to go through the details of his life by talking about how his symptom has affected his experiences in one way or another that is good therapeutic free association, and can be allowed to form even the bulk of the work done in the first four sessions. However, it will be far better if the equivalent of at least one session is allocated to other topics and memories.

In free association the therapist should only speak when he really has too. Ninety per cent of the time it is the client who: should be talking, while the therapist writes down, as best he can, all that is said.

There are many benefits in writing down what has been said:

One, almost always in the first few minutes the client will, without realising it, refer directly or indirectly to the cause of his problem, or at least give some clue.

Two, you have a visible record of what was said, and one that you can scan or look back to readily.

Three, you can read it, or part of it, back to him in a subsequent session, and help him pick up where he left off in the previous one. Another advantage is that you can mark off points of interest that might be important later.

Four, writing down what he says will keep you concentrating, because there could be little worse for the client/therapist relationship than your client talking away, only to find that you had let your mind wander and had not taken a word in for some time.

At all times be prepared with tissues and sympathy. Beware the unexpected question like:

"Should I divorce her?" You must always be non-committal. Being a hypnotherapist does not qualify you as a counsellor, advisor or adjudicator, nor do you want to spend time as a witness in divorce hearings. Tell them, should they seek such advice, that it is not for the therapist to advise or to judge, and that your job is to help them to get better so that they can make their own decision, but from a clearer mind.

Clients will often say: "I know I'm being silly" or "I know you'll think I'm being stupid" or "I know you think I've only myself to

RESOLVING SEXUAL ISSUES
with Creative Mindpower Techniques

blame". What they are really saying is, please reassure me, and please tell me you don't think I'm being silly. Respond to their need and reassure them. I often do this by saying that I certainly do not think they are being silly, but that they are being a bit hard on themselves considering what they have been through.

Keep in mind too, the unsympathetic conditions they will often have had to live with. This is their chance to be taken seriously, so give them their full opportunity to freely make the most of being with you. A sentence often occurring in the thank you letters I receive is along the lines of: "Throughout our sessions you never once judged me, you just listened with a caring and considerate manner".

Having completed the first session, de-induce hypnosis, following some gentle words of encouragement, especially praise them if they have done well.

If you have the confidence it is also helpful to make a post-hypnotic suggestion that "when you are here next time and I click my fingers with the command sleep you will instantly return to this deep, pleasant state of relaxation you are enjoying now, but *only* when *I* say sleep and *only* in this room" (this latter ensures the client does not go into hypnosis if someone else happens to say "sleep" – the client may well be driving at the time!)

Repeat the post-hypnotic suggestion three times then de-induce the client. This post hypnotic suggestion saves the time needed to induce hypnosis at the next session.

Dr. Frank W. Lea, DD,
Dip.NLP(Master Practitioner), RPHH, APHP

SESSION TWO (possibly 3 and 4)

Sessions two, three and four are, in principle, really just the continuation of the process of free association begun in the first session. But there are one or two points worth noting. Although the second session can occur even on the following day, subsequent sessions should be not less than five days apart, and any gap of more than two weeks should be avoided.

The 'same time next week' idea is best.

For most, particularly when clients start out well, sooner or later they are going to report having had a bad week, perhaps fearful that all the progress they thought they had made up until then had been an illusion. Following a 'down' week they may feel that their hopes are shattered, and become convinced they will never recover, whereas unknown to them, their set-back or bad week is an excellent sign of progress, though they are not likely to see it that way. In more cases than not, around session four, five or six, hope is at risk of abandonment by the client.

Although the client is too nice to say so, somewhere around the middle of his treatment sessions he will begin to think that the treatment isn't going to work for him; that he has not been hypnotised, or at least, not in the way he expected it, that he cannot see the connection between his treatment and his problem that everything he has told you he knew about already and that perhaps he's just not very good at it, or not responding somehow.

The good therapist will not only watch for the signs of all this, but if the signs do not show will take the bull by the horns and bring the matter up, and tell him how most people are feeling about now, mentioning the points above. If this is not done, do not be surprised if your client fails to appear around session five, or six. Especially should he begin to feel worse as his repression begins to surface.

Should he terminate his treatment he will have abandoned his attempt, abandoned you, and remain stuck with his problem, possibly in a worse form. In short, he hasn't failed you, you will have failed him.

Note: If a client is particularly responsive and doing well it is possible to skip sessions three or four or both and go on to session five. This relies on the good judgment of the therapist. If you do decide to skip a session the client will appreciate the fact that you are not charging him for more sessions than required and respect your honesty.

SESSION FIVE

In every session following the first, it is a sound practice to ask the client how they have been feeling during the previous week. Not only is this a courteous practice, but it keeps the therapist in touch with progress. Normally the client will reply in his social habit by saying he is "Fine", or the week has been "All right", adding "Thank you". This type of social response is not enough, the question is a medical one and some further details are required. In particular, it helps in dealing with the points raised earlier, when the client might terminate his treatment prematurely by thinking the sessions are failing. By session five an in-depth assessment of progress before commencing therapy is essential for additional reasons.

In session five, after inducing hypnosis, you are to report the progress, or lack of it, back to his subconscious as an important part of the work. After inducing hypnosis I say that since nineteen out of twenty clients will require eight sessions, I regard the fifth session rather as the beginning of the second-half of the treatment and as such, feel it is a good time to review progress. By now I have a good understanding of him he is feeling easy with me and has accepted me.

Having told him of my intention to sum up our progress I go through and emphasise, all the good points. For example, I may proceed as follows:

"In summing up my feelings as regards progress, I would like to make a few points. I can't put them in any order of importance, so I will just raise them as they come to mind." Firstly, however, there is one point that I would like to put on top of the list though. You know, when someone comes in here and asks me to help them with some important or vital aspect of their life, I feel tremendously flattered and I thank you for that flattery.

You see, I'm not just being asked to supply a loaf of bread, or produce something that will wear out. What I'm being asked to do is to change a person's quality of life, not just temporarily, but forever. It's a vitally important job and, as I say, thanks for flattering me by asking me to do it. "

"Secondly, I have asked you to work with me in a way that for many doesn't seem a likely route to success, even though it is. However, you've got on with it, and not just that, but you've done well and given me the sort of effort I need for my work and in quality too.

"Again, you've been interesting to work with; I have enjoyed your company and looked forward to seeing you each time. I respect your values; you've got a nice character. In short, I think you are what I choose to call a 'goodly human being

"Also, in this I see myself working for your children, wife, parents, and all the others in your life, for your friends and the people who work with you, because all of us are made that bit happier by coming into contact with someone who is confidently just getting on with life - just as we are that bit cast down when we come across someone down on his luck, or out of sorts. It's like dropping a stone in a pool, the ripples from our work spread out to the benefit of all. I have plenty of motivation to help you, the cause is wholly worthwhile and I thank you for that too."

<u>Note:</u> Whatever you do say has to be genuine, and from the heart, for if it is not the client will detect the insincerity. It may seem gushing or over the top, but if what you say is true the client will be flattered. On occasions he may even burst into tears, replying that nobody has ever spoken so nicely to him before.

In what follows next, good judgment is required. You are going to continue with firmness, directly related to what the client can be expected to accept without feeling overtaxed or driven too hard. With the psychologically frail or badly hurt client you will be very gentle. With those of a much harder mental make-up you will need to be *more* forceful, raising your voice and possibly emphasising your points in some way. In the illustration that follows, I present the more emphatic approach following limited progress.

Having given my praise, I deliberately pause to enabling him to respond or momentarily to take in what has just been said. If he does respond - his modesty will mostly restrict him - I curtail his response by what I say next. I continue: "However, there is another point I must add, a point that's far from as attractive as what I have just said.

There is something here that is far from satisfactory, something that must be faced too!" (Pause for a response which, if any, must be curtailed). Continuing I go on to say: "While you have been getting on with your work, while you've been doing all those things that I have just thanked and praised you for, I have to tell you that your subconscious has not been keeping pace with your efforts. It's been letting you down, for you do still have your problem, don't you?"

I await confirmation but curtail any response, then continue: "I say that your subconscious is hiding a very guilty secret, and I will justify that statement, for it has to be a secret in your subconscious, because you don't know what it is that is upsetting your mind and causing the problem do you?" (Response - and curtailed again)

"I say a guilty secret because that secret is upsetting you with the symptom - that must be true as well, mustn't it?" (Any response again curtailed) "You see, you don't get upset with having a secret of what you're going to give someone for Christmas, so your subconscious must have a guilty secret and that statement must be true too! I say the time has come for a vital decision to be made and in here today! I did say that I was flattered to be asked to help, and as such, I don't like your subconscious failing you and hindering me. I have no axe to grind with you, but your subconscious has not yet played its full part in helping you by resolving your problem, and by letting you know what its secret is."

"That's a failure of its duties to you, your subconscious should be co-operating with you helping you to feel far better. Now, I am going to ask your subconscious four questions, it does not have to answer them, but if it does choose to answer, let me add this too. I shall hold it to any response it makes, there will be no going back on its word, changing its stance or failing in the commitment to the answers it gives".

"Before I continue, do you understand the premise upon which I shall ask the questions? (Yes!) Good! Mind you, if your answers are negative or don't come, then I shall have to end our work, and, subconscious, I must point out to you, that if you do not co-operate, you will

take *(client's name)* away today to do the best you can, and can I remind you, your best hasn't done *(client's name)* problem much good lately".

"Okay, here's the first question. I say that there are two parts to your life, there's the past, and for all of your experiences, good bad and indifferent, the past is over and gone. On the other hand, there's your 'here-and-now' and the future, and you have to live through that. You can anticipate it, mould it, enjoy it and make the most of it.

Now I say that your subconscious should be concerning itself with perfecting the future and making the most of it, rather than being more concerned with the past. "

"So, subconscious, do you agree that your future is the most important part of your life now, and the part you should be concerned with and concentrating on?" ("Yes! ") "Good!

"So you choose to answer the questions, and of course, you are right. Let me emphasise the validity of your answer. I know of two psychotic patients, let's call them X and Y, who both do the same thing, for most of the day they sit on the floor, wrap their arms around their knees and bury their faces between their wrists. They will briefly acknowledge visitors, stop to eat, or go to the toilet, but other than that, that's how they spend their days."

"What's happening of course is that they have withdrawn, magnetised by some past events in their lives. I can't help them, but it does show how serious it can be to concentrate only upon the past. For them there is no here and now, nor any future!"

"Right, then would you also agree that if it is some past event that produced your guilty secret, and one that undermines your prospects for the future, that the matter should be brought to the surface, dealt with, and got out of the way?" ("Yes! ") "Good. Do you know how they produce a cultured pearl? Let me tell you. A grain of sand is inserted into the oyster, the oyster then proceeds, not to eject it, but to cover it up and hide it with mucus which we call pearl. Of course, it then becomes a greater problem because it has been enlarged"

"So, the oyster follows the same procedure as before, but as it does so the problem doesn't get resolved, but just keeps on getting bigger. Until eventually, the problem becomes so enlarged by the attempted faulty solution, that the oyster endures constant agony. Without going into the why of its reaction, it does demonstrate the folly of attempting to conceal a problem. What the oyster should have done of course was to have ejected that sand particle in the first place then it would not have suffered.

"So you agree that your future is more important to you than the past, and that any guilty secret from your past should be brought to the surface and be dealt with." "Good!"

"As valid as those two decisions are let us just move them aside for the moment and take up another issue for consideration, all by itself. I have had, people come in here with a wide range of medical and psychological conditions, and I have found that in the vast majority of cases that their conditions have been rooted in some guilty secret hidden in their minds. If by resolving your guilty secret you could ensure a longer, healthier and happier life would you agree that is a good enough reason to do so?" (Yes)

"Good. Then here is my fourth question, will you agree to do just that?" ("Yes! ") (Pause)

(Client's name) "I did say how much this work means to me as well as to you, didn't I? (Yes") Then you will understand that I can't take any chances. You see, I think your subconscious has held its guilty secret for years, and probably even longer than you've been aware of it. Yet your subconscious appears to have done nothing about resolving it, but in here, your subconscious only having known me for a few hours, appears to have made a great decision for change. Can you understand that I need to check that it really means what it has said? (Yes), "good, then I will check that right now".

"I am going to touch your index finger now", *(touch* "Subconscious, if you mean what I have heard you say, that you have had enough, and see all the benefits of resolving your guilty secret by letting *(client's name)* know what it is, then I want you to cause that finger to react by moving it now"

(Await the signal, and request it again if necessary. Ignore any movement that the client admits he has deliberately made.) The signal must be watched for carefully, because it might only be a small nerve reaction and may not be repeated if it is missed. Where no signal is detected the client should be asked if he felt one. Often the client will report that he did feel some sensation in his finger or hand, this indicates the subconscious has answered `yes`.

In the extremely unlikely situation where no such confirmation signal is transmitted, further negotiation with the subconscious is called for, especially to explore the possibility of some concealed motive. Personally I have never experienced such a situation.

However, confronted with such a unique outcome I would press on, hoping for the best, relying on the logic of what is to follow to override the subconscious's reluctance. All having gone well so far, as it usually does, with an open expression of pleasure I thank the client's subconscious.

AN ALTERNATIVE APPROACH TO SESSION FIVE

An alternative to the approach given before is used where it is judged appropriate, either because the client is still too psychologically frail or the client has already made significant progress. The praise is still given however, but followed by presenting the questions in a helpful, understanding caring way of reasoning, stressing more the simple logic of the benefits of change.

Where the client has already made significant progress, the questions are put forward more in the way of supporting continuing change, incorporating such statements as: "As you have already found out, such changes are welcome and beneficial", or "Your subconscious has already realised", or "Your subconscious has already commenced the process of change", or "Changes for the better are now coming faster and faster" and the like.

Note: The wording given is merely to give the student an idea of how to proceed, it is best if you use your own words.

SUMMING UP

In whatever form it takes, There are two reasons for conducting the first part of session five in the first way suggested.

The first is the benefit to the client, because the client's subconscious has been aware of its problem for some time, probably years, and has not only become used to having it, but by now considers it a normal state. However, the procedure has now focused the subconscious's attention on it in a new way, and the importance of resolving it has been stressed and accepted, and all this with the client in hypnosis, which is in itself a totally different state of mind to the one in which he has previously only consciously wished his problem would go away.

The benefit is further enhanced because by this session, his subconscious has accepted the therapist, it has been exercised and it has become more aware of the root cause of the problem anyway. Another benefit is for the therapist, for he is now going to be working on the basis that 'planning permission for change' has been given, and the need for it agreed. The therapist now has an enormously powerful argument, based upon logic and agreement that he can use should difficulties or resistance emerge later.

For instance, should the subconscious, not wishing to 'hurt' the client's conscious mind by releasing the cause of the problem to it, the therapist can remind it that it has agreed to release him, and confirmed its intention of doing so.

Quite often, in session seven, this powerful argument is used, and where it is it, is often the crucial point that finally releases the repression.

PART TWO OF SESSION FIVE

This and session six can be a very effective method that you can use for yourself as a means of contacting your own subconscious in order to resolve problems or issues.

Following the successful conclusion to the first part of this session, I invite the subconscious to begin (or continue to) the release of the problem(s) by using the exercise to follow.

I continue "Now I want you to build a picture in your mind, I want you to imagine that you are going on a trip to meet a very wise old man, who lives in a cave on a mountain. (On occasions female clients, but rarely males, will prefer a wise old woman. Such a choice is perfectly acceptable.) You have started your journey and at the moment, have paused on the mountain track. From where you are the track slopes gently upwards. It's midnight, but above is the biggest and brightest moon that you have ever seen. There's no movement in the air and the temperature is perfect.

Wafting up from the valley below is the wonderful aroma of the pine trees, blending with the scent of the wild mountain flowers on the slopes. Say 'yes' when you are there in the picture." ("Yes! ") "Good."

"Now I want you to begin moving forward, as you go look for two large boulders, between which a soft green grass path leads off to one side, turn onto the path and say 'yes' when you have." ("Yes! ") "Good, feel the soft grass underfoot, see the mountain flowers in it, their colours, like the grass, all changed by the light from the moon.

Gone are the pinks, reds and yellows, now the flowers are white, grey and black, and the grass is a deep olive. Shortly, ahead of you among the few trees on this part of the mountain, you will see the occasional flicker of flame that comes from the dying embers of the wise old man's camp fire of the day. Say 'yes' when you see them. ("Yes!") "Good".

"The grass path curves and leads you down a shallow slope and out into a small clearing. Over there is the wise old man's camp fire. See the orange red glow of the burning timbers, the brilliant white of the ash, and see too that thin strand of white smoke gently rising into the air *(pause)* and there beside the fire is a pile of logs, and over there is the entrance to the cave itself. Now go forward and pick up four or five of the logs and drop them into the fire so that the fire crackles and flares up so brightly that, by the light of those dancing flames you can see inside the cave itself. "

"Tell me what it looks like in there?" *(Response)* "Good. Now shortly, coming towards you from the back of the cave, the wise old man will move forward to greet you. As he comes forward describe him for me, what does he wear, what's on his feet, does he have a beard?" *(Client describes)* "Now, as he greets you I'm going to ask him some questions. He may answer in many ways, he may smile, shrug his shoulders make some gesture with his hands, nod or shake his head, wink or say something. What I want you to do is to tell me what he means by his reactions".

I then proceed with the questions. "Wise old man, is it possible for *(client's name)* to be released from his problem?" (Expect 'Yes', if 'No' *(rare indeed)* the present wise old man is a fraudster, and should be sent back to be replaced by the genuine one, and the question repeated.) "Then, wise old man, since it is possible for *(client's name)* to be freed from his condition, would you agree to use all your wisdom and efforts to help *(client's name)* do so?" ("Yes!") "Good. Then, wise old man, with my experience and knowledge helping him will *(Client)* get better? (Yes) "Good"

"Wise old man, *(client's name)* may need you and your help at any time in the future, to inspire him, to help him with important decisions and the like. If *(client's name)* finds that he needs that help, would you come forward and give it?" ("Yes! ") "Good. Suddenly there is a 'crack' from the fire, causing you to look at it. You see a small jet of violet-blue flame rising from the fire; tell me when you see it" (Yes).

"See how beautiful it looks, but now as you return your gaze to the wise old man, you see him offering you a present - what is he giving you?" *(Response).* "The time has come for you to leave, I want you to say farewell to the wise old man and go back along the path to the two boulders and tell me when you are there". (Here) "Good"

I then discuss the present the wise old man has given. Mostly it will be symbolic but it will always have a positive meaning. A book say, either with instructions for a better life, or empty to symbolize the freedom to write a new life. It may be a diamond or a gold bar to represent good-will and fortune in some way, a torch, to help light up life in future, or a walking stick to help him on his passage ahead, a parcel, either empty, signifying his problems are to be gone, or the parcel might contain something, perhaps some mess representing his problems are given to him for him to throw away. Whatever the gift, there will be a positive meaning which should be looked for.

For example, one client was given a shiny piece of coal which she realised that where she originally came from a piece of coal meant good luck. The gift will often be something that reminds the client of a time when he felt good, happy or positive.

Next, following a short discussion of the present, I ask who the wise old man is. Many will answer, 'Jesus' or 'Merlin' their grandfather and so on, but sometimes they will guess the truth, that he is their subconscious. The wise old man exercise is, without the client consciously realising it, bringing the conscious and subconscious minds into contact with each other, using the subconscious's natural interpretation methods, and confirming the commitment to change.

In conclusion, in three separate ways, the subconscious has said 'yes' to his willingness to resolve his problems. The purpose in both parts of session five has been to significantly exercise his mind and concentrate it on bringing about change. Of course, he has also been prompted by previous case histories, illustrating the benefits of doing so. Significant subconscious activity can now be expected in the client. During the coming week he may well hit a 'bad-patch' as the root cause of his problem does begin to surface.

SESSION SIX

NEURO LINGUISTIC PROGRAMMING. (NLP)

With some clients, N.L.P. will cause little if any significant reactions, but in many it will. In about one-in-five cases these reaction can also be intensely emotional. N.L.P. can be compared to a directed dream experience, but carried out in hypnosis rather than sleep, with the conscious mind making a significant contribution to the process.

Amazing improvements can follow it, sometimes instantly too. It is particularly relevant where the client has been a significant victim of one of the Oedipus or Elecra complex. It can also be useful with clients that have had a difficult childhood, a past relationship problem or in coming to terms with the loss of a loved one. During the process the subconscious is drawn to matters that concern it, and in conjunction with the conscious mind attempts to resolve them and in so doing mostly succeeds.

To begin the process I usually remind the client that in session five we imagined visiting the wise old man, and say that I want to go through a similar exercise again. I tell the client though that I want him to explore his own mind, and since I can't expect him to imagine himself clambering through a lot of assorted grey material, I shall ask him to imagine that his mind is made up of rooms, corridors, cupboards and the like, rather:- like an office. I then continue: "So to begin with, imagine you are just standing in a lovely broad corridor, well lit and wonderfully decorated. Say 'yes' when you are there". (Yes!)

Note: Occasionally a client may have, at first, some difficulty at attempting this. If he does encourage him and if he should find continuing difficulties it is most likely to be because the explanation of the complex is still seriously distracting his subconscious, particularly if he managed the previous visit to the wise old man easily. As such, it is a good sign that you were right in putting the concept forward. You may, in cases where the inability to imagine the scene continues, return to free association or take up some other issue, because in such cases his mind is still too busy to concentrate on imaginative things.

Assuming the client, as most do, goes along with the requested imagining by responding with that 'yes', continue: "Good, now I want you to become aware that you are standing on one of the most luxurious carpets you've ever walked on, so look down and tell me, what colour or colours it is made of?" Often he will say red, meaning that his subconscious feels anger or determination.

Alternative colours can mean other feelings: brown, subconsciously feeling messy; blue, I feel good, relieved, or want to feel good; yellow, I am looking for or expecting a new beginning, a fresh start; green, I feel optimistic; grey, I am feeling neutral; purple, there is a sexual matter that bothers me; pink, I'm thinking of my mother, or with the female client, "I'm female and proud of it". No colours can be taken as hard fact, but you will have at least a possible guide to the client's feelings.

Having received the colour answer, I then invite the client to begin to move down the corridor until he reaches a door, and that when he can see it he should again say 'yes'. (Yes!) "Good! Now through that door is a room that contains all the units which control every aspect of your body and mind. Those units may appear as computer terminals, filing cabinets, cupboards or control panels. Now I want you to enter and describe what you see". *(Client describes)* "Good! Now, are there any warning lights or any other indications that show anything to be wrong or not working properly?"

If the client says 'No', get him to check again, but do not suggest that you expected warning lights or signals. If 'No' again, proceed with part B below. If your client reports such a light, lights or signals, ask him to go over to it or to the nearest one if there are two or more, and tell you what that unit controls or does for him. He may not know what that unit does for him, but more often he will have some idea.

For example, a lady client finding such a warning light said the unit looked after her hair, and commented that she had been very worried about a serious recent hair loss. She imagined herself rectifying the unit, and the fault indicating light going off when she had done so. She was to ring me, several weeks after her treatment, to say her home hairdresser had just asked her what she had used to restore her hair to such luxurious healthy growth.

Where a fault indicating light or signal is reported, next ask what is wrong with the unit. If they don't know, suggest a computer disc may be jammed, some wire could be loose, or that the unit is not tuned in properly or make similar suggestions. Encourage them to find the fault and then to remedy it in some way - even to replacing the unit if needs be.

If they encounter some difficulty ask them to look for an internal telephone. When they have found it, ask them to ring for the wise old man and to tell you when he's arrived. In this approach, when your client says the wise old man is there, tell your client to indicate the problem to him, and to watch as he carries out the repairs until the warning light or signal goes off. Repeat similar exercises for any other fault indications, either with or without the wise old man, according to whether he has been sent for or not. This procedure, which sometimes seems just like a game to the client, can have amazing effects, for in it you are using the subconscious's natural healing methods.

PART 'B'

Any such fault indications having been dealt with, continue but now in an almost apprehensive or concerned sort of voice, thus: "Now, somewhere in that room is another door, not the one you came in by, but another. Say yes when you see it. (Yes!) Now in a moment, not yet, I will ask you to cross the room and go through that door, closing it behind you, and when you have, stand rigidly still with your back to the door and say yes when you are there. Please do that now". (Yes!) Next continue" speaking more slowly and softly, with the approach being intended to heighten the intensity and expectation of the client.

"Look slowly around the room and tell me, is there somebody already in there? (If No) Look around again, look for any shadow that might mean someone hiding behind a pillar, curtain or cupboard". If no indication of another person initially results, persist a little longer, or continue by saying, "Okay, since this is your mind, we can think of this room as your managing director's office, and in that case, there is an adjacent room to this one that is used for people waiting to set you. Tell me when you can see the door that leads to that room". (Yes!) Having come this far, a No is most unlikely. "Good, then go in there and tell me who is waiting for you".

Note: Sooner or later the client, in most cases, will find someone or some people. These will be those who either are, or have been important to them in some way, and most often they will fit into one of four broad categories. One: their current love, and following the complex explanation, this will signify their freedom to love them. Two: someone who has caused them harm. Three: relatives or parents, or the parent of the opposite sex, again often a complex related imagery, or Four: a deceased family relative or friend.

The variations, feelings, reactions and experiences are so many that only an idea of what the therapist is to have his client do can be given here. In essence the event has to be of a constructive positive nature, making up, embracing, forgiving and the like. Where the attempt to release any animosity fails, ask the client to tell the person to leave and watch him go. He should see himself tell that person to go in a controlled positive way. Commonly there will be tears, of a happy, sad, or angry nature.

When the exercise is completed in the managing director's office or the waiting room, ask your client to go back to his control-room, and when he has arrived, to say if any new warning signal has come on while he's been busy out of the room. If 'Yes', proceed as earlier, or if 'No', as it mostly will be, ask him to return to the corridor and say 'yes' when he is there. ('Yes!) "Now I want you to realise that while you have been doing your work, the carpet fitters have been in and laid a brand-new carpet, look down at it, and tell me what colour or colours do you see now."

The colours will again portray his subconscious feelings. If you have been conscientious in your work, and used an underlying tone of enthusiasm in dealing with whatever situations may have arisen, you will have brought about positive changes, though you may not be able to name those changes, they are most likely to be reflected in the colour or colours to be reported to you in the new carpet. Hope above all, for yellow and more especially gold, meaning I see new opportunities and/or a fresh start, or green for optimism and blue for feeling good.

SESSION SEVEN

By this time most clients will mostly report feeling better in some way they may even be boastful of their recent personal achievements, now being freer of their previous symptoms and possibly they may dismiss, out of hand, any interest in some previous symptom, and now regarding it as irrelevant. Most will have come a long way from the original starting point they presented to you at your first meeting, but expect about one-in-five to report little if any progress though. While this is naturally disappointing to both, when such negative reports are made at this stage take heart, for you have a session seven 'tool kit' that hasn't even been used yet.

Here's how to proceed. Take the client into hypnosis, and deepen this into the somnambulistic state. Get him to help you draw up a statement representing his most important outstanding requirements, one that you can read back to his subconscious. An example statement might be as follows:

"Subconscious, Harry reports to me that he continues to suffer agony with his migraine, and that this agony is ruining his life.

Further, subconscious, Harry reports that his social life is ruined and that he can no longer concentrate on his work. Subconscious, Harry desperately needs to be released from his awful condition, and asks that you release him and in here today. Subconscious, you know what it is that occurred in Harry's life and caused his migraine and his suffering, Harry wants you to return to that incident, that original experience, and pass the memory of it back to him. Subconscious this is an easy and simple thing for you to do. Focus in on that memory clearly, so that when shortly I count to three and click my fingers, you do pass that memory to him.

"Subconscious I will read this statement to you twice more, as you get ready to do so". (*Read the statement twice more*) Then say to the client: "You are going back Harry, back to a time when the event that caused your migraine actually occurred, or to a time it is just about to occur". (*Be positive and confident - this is going to happen, just as you* say *it will*) "One, two, three 'click'!". (A moment's pause), then prompt with such questions as: "Are you inside or out?" "Is anyone with you?" "What's happening now?" "How do you feel?

Around fifty to sixty percent of such cases will immediately produce the abreaction required, producing the sort of result given in the case histories quoted. The client may report being aware of some feeling, or see something that doesn't make sense.

Unless the abreaction, in mostly an emotive state, comes out in full, further prompting may be needed such as: "Subconscious, I will count to three and again click my fingers and you add to that memory (or feelings) you have just had, with something else, but always coming nearer and nearer to the actual moment that led to Harry's awful migraine".

If, after several attempts you have been unsuccessful, there are other tools in your session seven kit that you can then use. Don't forget the agreement reached in session five, and remind his subconscious that it did agree to bring about change and that you know that the agreement will be honoured. The following method could also be used.

"Subconscious, Harry desperately needs you to release him from his awful migraine, and you may do so in any way you feel most appropriate. You may release him by causing him to have some feeling, like causing him to feel he is floating, feeling as if he is spinning, being pushed back into the chair, tipping sideways or some other sensation. You may have him feeling himself going down a tunnel, and out into the light, by just throwing the emotion to the surface, or giving him that memory or a thought. When I count to three and click my fingers subconscious, you carry out that release, and in any manner appropriate. One, two, three 'click'!"

With a little patience, and using these methods in various combinations, nine out of ten clients will have responded or will have begun to. Using your initiative you may further encourage the client, saying such things as: "It is coming through, you are getting there, your subconscious is recalling and releasing the event", etc. Don't rush your client and above all, remain positive and patient. Should you continue to experience difficulties, tell your client you are going to take another issue or symptom, should there be one, while his subconscious continues to release, in this case, his migraine.

There will often be something else. Where there is another symptom or issue, there is no real need to write a second statement, since the client's subconscious will understand the principle by then. Because of this, an unscripted repetition of an approach similar to the original one can now be expected to bring the desired result. Sometimes a secondary issue will not only be successful in its own right, but directly lead to a successful outcome of the first attempt.

Conversely, having gained a first abreaction, you may well be amazed at the simple ease with which other issues or symptoms release themselves. With abreaction's now coming one after the other until, if there are say, four or five on your list, some may even be released upon merely being mentioned. My personal record is eight in a row. Abreaction releases and memories just popping up in just a few minutes, while I had spent half an hour releasing the first.

Following this session, often the most productive, revealing and satisfying one, expect your client to feel mentally drained. If he is, that's an excellent technical sign of good progress. Despite any doubts of success you may initially have had, session seven is likely to demonstrate most effectively the enormous healing powers of hypnotherapy, to your client, any attending guest, and not least to yourself, a magnificently satisfying experience to all.

FINAL WORDS

In these writings, only a tiny fraction of my experiences have been illustrated and some, with a great feeling of immense personal satisfaction, will live with me forever, and what I have done, starting from scratch, you can do too if you decide to study further and become a professional therapist.

It is my sincere hope that this little book helps even just a few people to understand themselves and overcome any sexual problems or issues they may have.

Those who wish to deal with other psychological and issues such as stress, anxiety and phobias or physiological conditions such as PMT, IBS, arthritis, psoriasis etc. will find all the knowledge and techniques in the sister book `Creative Mindpower Techniques to Heal Yourself and Others`

CONTACT THE AUTHOR

Should you wish clarification on any aspect of the book please feel free to contact the author by e-mail as below.

To become a Certified Practitioner of Creative Mindpower Techniques the reader would benefit from a two day practical training workshop for practice and demonstrations of the techniques. Contact the author for details.

If you have sexual issues or problems you wish to address, the sister book Creative Mindpower Techniques for Resolving Sexual Issues is especially written for this purpose.

THE AUTHOR IS AVAILABLE FOR
Private Therapy
Speaking Engagements
Talks and Practical Demonstrations
Media Interviews and Magazine Articles.

E-mail: actpublications@yahoo.co.uk

www.ingramcontent.com/pod-product-compliance
Lightning Source LLC
Chambersburg PA
CBHW021604280526
45784CB00001BA/497